D0873339

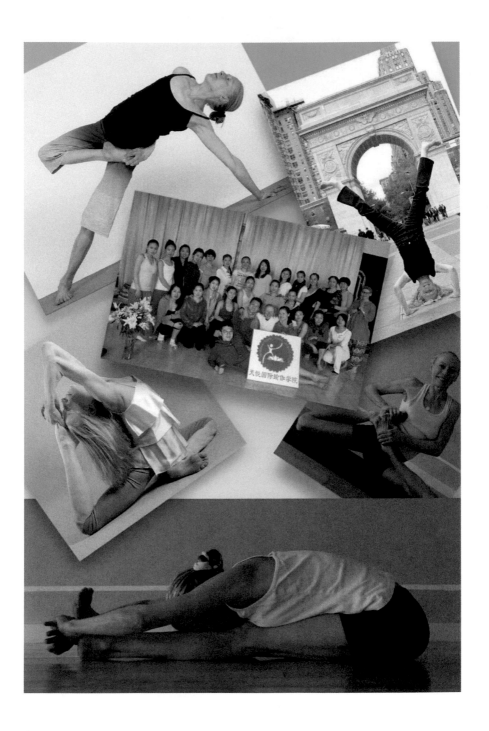

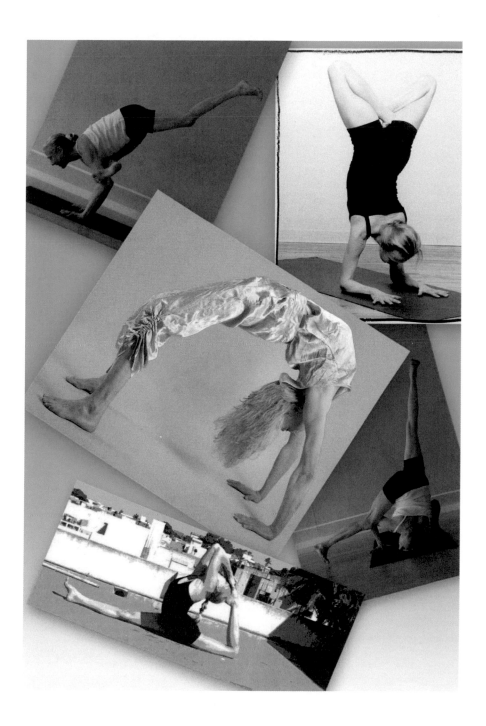

# HIP OP
# Beyond Recovery

ISBN-13: 978-1-7334185-0-8
In Print Publications

# HIP OP:
# Beyond Recovery

Lois Nesbitt, Ph.D., E-RYT 500

"In this engaging, witty, and honest book, Lois Nesbitt walks us through the challenges of a failing hip and the path to a miraculous recovery.  This is a book full of good advice, personal narrative, and philosophy, one that anybody contemplating a major life challenge would do well to read.  It is a contemplation of what it means to heal."

—Andrew Solomon, National Book Award-winning author of *Far from the Tree* and *The Noonday Demon*

"Lois Nesbitt's journey of healing her body is sheer inspiration. After 25 years of exploration as a teacher of teachers, she offers us ways to come out of any dark time with honesty, humility, and gratitude"

—Elena Brower, bestselling author of *Practice You* and *Art of Attention*

"Lois shows us the way to surrender to our worst fear and how freeing this is. Those facing major challenges including joint and structural problems of all sorts will find her words valuable. People with healthy bodies can also learn how to move through the darkness toward the light!"

—Richard P. Brown, M.D., Associate Clinical Professor of Psychiatry at Columbia University and creator of  *BREATH-BODY-MIND™ integrative healing*.

*What thou lovest well remains,*
*the rest is dross*
*What thou lov'st well shall not be reft from thee*

*—Ezra Pound, "Canto LXXXI"*

*You're in pretty good shape for the shape you're in*

*—Dr. Seuss*

## ACKNOWLEDGMENTS

It does indeed take a village, sometimes more than one. Many thanks to:

- My parents, who loved the idea of this book enough to read through and comment on countless drafts, as well as talking over every twist and turn of the process, while never suggesting there might be better uses of my time
- My siblings, Kate and Ralph, who always have my back, my hip, and every other part of me
- My longtime friend and guide Janet Nolan, who was there for me before, during, and after, pre- and post-op, as she always has been
- My assistants Sayaka Kubo, who got this project off the ground and contributed many of the photographs, and Jason Leek, who swept in to finish the job with great finesse
- Ed Gifford, who filmed the video for my crowd-funding campaign
- My friend and student Marian Robinson, who lent her considerable publishing expertise (and that of her colleagues) freely and enthusiastically to each stage of the project conception and development; and Paul Gordon, who designed the eye-catching cover
- Friends who guided me toward and through surgery: Peter Turino, Beverley Murphy, Camille Patrillo, Shig Ogyu, James Chew, my housemates Andy Stenerson, Katy Brennan, and Jennifer Corazzo, and the legions of 12-step recovery fellows who of course remain anonymous
- The communities at the yoga studios I taught: Jessica Bellofatto and the students, teachers, and trainees of KamaDeva Yoga; Jolie Parcher and the students and teachers at Mandala Yoga; and Erica Velasquez at Yoga in the Vines
- The nameless angels who carried my bags, helped me up and down stairs, or offered me a seat
- Medical professionals: My surgeon, Dr. David Mayman, and the staff of the Hospital for Special Surgery in New York City; Dr. Patrick Meere, Dr. Roy Davidovitch, and Dr. Stephen Honig at NYU Langone; Dr. Richard Brown; Dominque Richard; Alex Morales (PT), and massage therapists Tim Delonay and Liza Adara
- My yoga teachers: John Friend, founder of Anusara Yoga; Prof. Douglas Brooks, of the University of Rochester and Rajanaka Yoga; Leslie Kaminoff; Eddie Stern and John Campbell of the Patanjali Yoga Shala; Sharon Gannon and David Life of Jivamukti Yoga; and Swami Ramananda of Integral Yoga Institute
- All of the wonderfully generous contributors to my Indiegogo crowd-funding campaign
- The many, many students who have lit up my life for the past 25 years
- The extraordinary teachers at Harvard and Princeton who taught me the value of a word well spoken and a story well told

# Table of Contents

CHAPTER ONE

# WHA' HAPPENED? FROM ACROBAT TO INVALID

*Often the worst thing that happens to us turns out to be the best.*

*—Anonymous*

*When you hit bottom, the only way to go is up!*

*—Anonymous*

Every story begins with . . . a story. Here's mine. While you might be tempted to skip over this in search of practical information that *you* can use, everything I have to share on that front springs from my own experience. Context is everything. So I'm jumping in with the hip problem, *my* hip problem, the focus of this book. In Chapter 3 I'll give you some backstory on the many factors and lifestyle "choices" that likely ended me up in the OR. Please don't skip that chapter either, as, being human, I'm guessing my choices are not that different from many of yours. And I urge you to turn that ship around while there's still time.

My hip problem, like most big problems, started small. A twinge, sometimes a prolonged ache, in my right buttock. Occasional, then gradual, then gradually worse, then really bad. Heard the parable about frogs? If you toss them into a pot of boiling water, they will immediately sense danger and jump out. If you leave them in a pot of gradually warming water, they will stay there till they die. They just don't notice gradual discomfort becoming dangerous.

I was a frog who stayed in the pot. Let it be said that I don't love complications. I find life often more than I can handle on a good day. I always seem to be slipping behind on something, neglecting something else entirely—procrastinating. I even had an idea for an autobiography called *I'm Behind . . . I'm So Behind!* To which one of my witty housemates replied, "Sounds like a book that will never get written." Point taken, as this hip book is now 3.5 years behind schedule.

So, as hard as it is to ignore physical pain, my first and most enduring response was, "I don't have time for this." It's a coping mechanism that I must have developed years ago to enable me to leapfrog (what's with the frogs today?) over things that probably deserve attention. Like the ankle I mangled falling off a curb in India, or the kneecap I pounded on a marble staircase during grad school at Princeton. Or unresolved tensions with housemates, professors, employers, or family members—simmerings that boiled over later and required a *lot* of time to patch up. A friend of mine used to say she had two feelings, "fine" and "busy." Worked for me—until it didn't.

Whereas a better adjusted person would probably have booked a doctor's appointment, I just kept hoping the pain would go away. Being an active person, I've "worked through" a host of other pains and come out the other end intact, through some combination of backing off certain activities, getting lots of high-quality bodywork, downing bottles of Aleve, and summoning large doses of hope.

I also know enough about the body to know that while joint pain commonly ends in surgery, there's not a lot doctors can do about most muscle pain. And since my pain was in the muscles of my butt, nowhere near the hip joint itself, I figured I had just overworked something that needed a rest. I've since learned about "referred pain," which happens when you feel discomfort in one place when the cause is ground zero.

So there I was, gradually warming frog in a pot, preferring, however unconsciously, slow death, prolonged discomfort beyond all reason, thinking the whole thing would just go away. Well, it didn't, and after about a year and a half of "warm" water, things got really hot. I found myself in excruciating, debilitating, 24/7 pain.

The whole thing started during my beloved barre fitness classes (based on ballet, yoga, and a mashup of classic resistance training), to which I had become rather addicted. As much as I hated the classes for being insurmountably tough, I had grown used to the familiar formula. Blue carpet, black socks, playground balls and exercise mats, mirrors everywhere. I'm no fan of loud music and teachers who yell at you through wireless microphones (confusing because the sound of their voices comes out of corner speakers, so you can never sense where they are in the room), but I enjoyed being told exactly what to do for each second of one hour each day. Being self-employed and hence self-governing, I find the constant need to prioritize exhausting. While in barre class, Simon said, and I did.

Indeed, my almost daily appearances at the studio provided a kind of stability in my otherwise routine-free life. Adult daycare, if you will. Fifty-seven predictable minutes filling in the gaps between my structured activities—time otherwise so easily frittered away by the self-employed. A high-performing crutch that not only accounted for my time but staved off midday loneliness. So, I was loath to accept that anything I did there might be causing me harm. I was

13

convinced the classes were providing the perfect complement to my yoga practice—which in many ways they were. I developed a stronger core (couldn't do three sit-ups at the first class!). I got stronger biceps, pecs, and quads, muscles oddly underused in yoga. Most of all, I got humble, being pretty much the worst student in the room for many months. I'm in my comfort zone when excelling at whatever it is I've taken on, so I gravitate to whatever comes easily and avoid the rest. I became a swimmer, a pianist, a visual artist, and a straight-A student because I sucked at kickball, basketball, volleyball, field hockey, and every other team sport. Being a serious student putting in lots of solitary hours doing homework justified not joining anything. I found organized groups tedious, fractious, or both. Plus, there were always people involved.

So, it was big shift to find myself in the remedial barre section after years of being the most advanced yogini in any class I took. Perhaps this voluntary humility cracked open the shell that would allow me to turn myself over to the doctors and physical therapists who knew a bit more about hip repairs than I. I do know that I learned to surrender to someone else's pacing and demands—often almost on the verge of tears when the teacher asked us to do one more rep on my already shaky, spindly legs.

Yet it got to the point that every time I rotated my leg in or out when my hip was flexed, which was often in those classes, I got this sharp, icky pain that eventually followed me home and kept me up at night. Then the same pain (along with another one, which migrated around to the front of my hip) started to haunt my yoga practice and teaching. Basically, any time I raised my leg toward my torso (like, when walking!), this new ache chimed in.

Alarm bells were going off. At some level I knew my ship was sinking. Mortality had yet to rear its monstrous head in my life to such a degree that I often forgot how old I was—and I mean by *decades*. When well into my thirties someone once asked me how old I was, and without thinking I replied, "19." Sounded weird even to me, but I had no intention to deceive. That's honestly how old I thought I was at that moment. Even today, without having kids and having sidestepped the standard markers of adult life—job, marriage, house, family—and having been blessed with two relatively spry parents pushing 90, I glide through life with the fresh idealism of a young child. Time is irrelevant. So, any signs that I might be infirm, wearing down, or *mortal* cause a logjam in my mind, what they call "cognitive dissonance."

But here I was, trying to assimilate debilitating sensations that seemed to have colonized my youthful body. In both barre and yoga, I started eliminating

14

troubling movements, hoping to reduce/remove the pain. I have a good grip on how our major muscles work, and I spend large parts of my days guiding others in how to move safely and effectively.

Along with avoiding what hurt, I tried giving myself physical therapy, a combo of stretching and strengthening the muscles I'd identified as the culprits (Gluteus Medius, Gluteus Minimus, Piriformis, and the tendon of the Rectus Femoris).

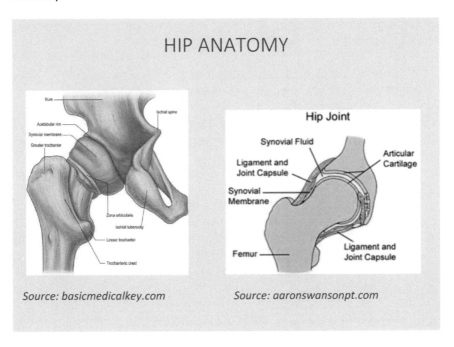

Source: basicmedicalkey.com                Source: aaronswansonpt.com

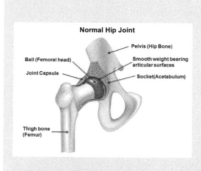

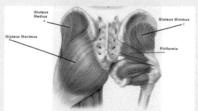

Source: dochenstyletaichi.com        Source: corewalking.com

## "THE THIGH BONE'S CONNECTED TO THE HIP BONE . . ."

Like the old song says, every bone in the body connects to some other bone (except the hyoid bone in the neck, far from our area of interest). Some fit together snugly, like spoons in a drawer or plates stacked on a shelf. Others not so much, like picking up random pieces of a model airplane kit and trying to get them to hold together with slow-drying glue. The hip is a good fit, a deep ball-and-socket joint, meaning lots of stability, but limited mobility. Which serves its specific purposes in your overall frame:

- Load-bearing: the entire weight of your torso, neck, head, and arms rests on your hip sockets
- Mobility: the top of the thighbone can rotate within its socket to allow you to sit, stand, walk, run, tango, leap over tall buildings . . .

The hip joint is held together by a network of ligaments (strings that tie bone to bone), tendons (which attach muscle to bone), and muscles, as well as the "joint capsule," a cuff that encloses the space between the top of the thigh bone (head of the femur) and the hip socket (acetabulum).

A ring of cartilage (soft tissue) between the head of the humerus and the socket provides padding, keeping the bones from rubbing against each other as you move around or simply compress the joint by sitting or standing up.

# HIP TROUBLE

The cartilage in all your joints is subject to wear and tear as you stumble along life's rocky path. If you don't stand and move in perfect alignment (and I've never seen a human do so), you're doing harm on a daily basis—and very possibly at this exact moment!

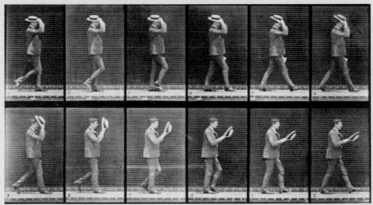

*Source: 1000museums.com*

Add to this any repetitive, stress- ("load")-inducing activities like serving a tennis ball, kicking a soccer ball, running a marathon or triathlon, vacuuming, shoveling snow, driving long distances, gardening, woodworking, and just about any other imaginable physical activity, and you've done some additional damage to the cartilage in various joints.

As we age, our bodies also dry out. No matter how much water you drink, your body doesn't retain it as well, and cartilage goes from feeling like a sponge saturated with water to one that sat dry on your kitchen counter for a week.

This dehydration also affects your muscles, tendons, and ligaments, making everything less elastic and thus less mobile. So even if the bones were a good fit to start with, you may no longer be able to get things back where they belong. (Think of "hunchbacks," whose upper bodies eventually get stuck rounded forward.)

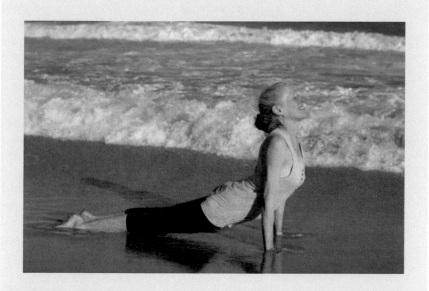

Think of our bodies as growing and maturing like plants. Young saplings are soft, moist, and malleable—often with an almost dangerous range of motion. Easily uprooted by strong winds or storm surges. Old trees are rigid and strong but brittle—fine until they snap. You too can expect to grow stiffer as you age. Still, that doesn't mean you've won a must-visit ticket to the OR. Depending on the luck of the gene draw, your past and present physical activities, your expectations of long-term strength and mobility, and how long you live, you may well sail through life on your God-given hips. Most people do. Studies estimate that .86% of the U.S. population has Total Hip Replacements, though the numbers increase with age (to some 6% among those over 80 years old). One trend worth noting: the number of middle-aged and younger people having hip replacements more than doubled in a recent decade—due perhaps in large part to our overall increase in athletic activity.

The numbers may seem small. On the other hand . . .

I also got lots of massage and bodywork from people I trust. My go-to, fellow anatomy geek and massage therapist, suggested I roll around on a

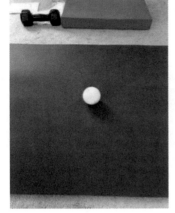

lacrosse ball whenever the pain kicked in. This turned out to be pure genius, more effective than massage, and infinitely cheaper and convenient. That trusty ball saw me through it all and found its place in my overnight bag when I finally went in for surgery. In fact, I still carry one around, figuring either I or any of my yoga students might need it when some muscle starts acting up. At $1.99 a pop, it's no problem that the dozens of such balls I've bought from Amazon have migrated into the hands of others or rolled to rest among the dust bunnies under furniture.

# CHAPTER TWO

## REALITY CHECK

*Pozzo: Give me that! (He snatches the hat from Vladimir, throws it on the ground, tramples on it.) There's an end to his thinking!*
*Vladimir: But will he be able to walk*
*Pozzo: Walk or crawl!*

—*Samuel Beckett, Waiting for Godot*

In the long run, my way didn't work. By December 2013, I was having pain just walking. Getting around New York City to teach my classes, buy groceries, run errands, visit doctors, whatever was increasingly problematic. Often I just stopped moving altogether, pausing mid-block as though expecting I

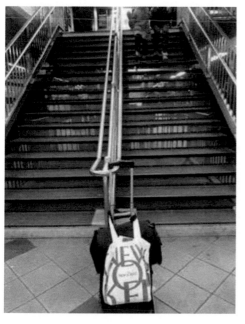

would somehow be magically airlifted to my destination. Subways were evil because climbing stairs hurt way more than just walking. People were stopping to ask if I needed help.

Sensing that I was out of my depth, I finally scheduled an appointment with a rheumatologist. My dad, a doctor, suggested that I start there before moving on to orthopedic surgeons, who might be too eager to suggest surgery. I liked the guy. We had a nice rapport. He patiently answered my questions and listened to my own theories about what was amiss. He moved my hip internally, externally, in and out of flexion, and just about every other way possible. Based on my range of motion (ROM) he said no chance of arthritis—good news! And since my gut feeling was that the problem was muscular, I happily concurred.

Yet the pain was real. The doctor explained that before my health insurance would sponsor an MRI (a pricey scan of soft tissues like muscles, tendons, and ligaments), we had to do the prerequisite x-rays, even though we both concurred that the issue was not arthritis, which affects bones.

# WHAT'S AN X-RAY? WHAT'S AN MRI?

## X-RAYS

If you've got intractable hip trouble, or persistent pain in any joint, your doctors are probably going to submit you to some high-tech observation—the kind that can't be done by watching you move or manually moving your limbs around in space to test your range of motion.

X-rays come first, for two reasons: they're relatively cheap (i.e., insurance will cover the cost), and they provide reliable images of your bones. And since a joint is a place where two or more bones meet, any joint diagnosis has to start by knowing how your bones are fitting together.

X-rays are quick and painless. X-ray beams pass through your body. The images produced indicate different types of tissue:
- Bones, the most dense, appear white
- The air in your lungs is black
- Fat and muscle are shades of gray.

(see photos, pp 26, 28)

Doctors will tell you that the amount of radiation exposure during X-rays is generally harmless, but notice how they always leave the room before the rays starting emitting! And they'll be careful to cover any sensitive parts of your anatomy with heavy radiation-prevention blankets.

# MRIS

Magnetic resonance imaging (MRI) uses a magnetic field and radio waves to create detailed images of organs and soft tissue (muscles, tendons, ligaments, cartilage). In most cases, you're inserted horizontally into a coffin-sized tube, within which the machine creates a magnetic field that temporarily realigns hydrogen atoms in your body. (One can only hope they remember to return "home" when it's all over!) Radio waves then cause the aligned atoms to produce faint signals, which are used to create cross-section images. MRIs can also produce three-dimensional images that can be viewed from many angles.

An MRI can reveal damaged tissues without the need to cut you open. That said, the cross-sections can't recreate a perfect image of your insides. Often surgeons don't get the full picture until you're in the OR, but it does give them something to go on before it comes to that.

MRIs don't carry any risk of radiation, but claustrophobics may find the procedure terrifying, as you have to remain in a relatively confined space, without moving, for up to an hour. Plus the machine makes all manner of humming, thrumming, banging, and clanging noises. High-end facilities will offer you a headset to listen to music that never quite blocks out the sound. Others will provide earplugs. But aside from the slightly unnerving images of your atoms being rearranged, MRIs are considered the standard non-invasive diagnostic tool for many injuries and ailments. Alas, they're much pricier than X-rays and usually involve some fancy footwork by your doctor's back-office staff to ensure that your insurance will cover the deed.

# OSTEO OR RHEUMATOID?
# ARTHRITIS FOR EVERYONE!

I should note here that there are two kinds of arthritis.

## TWO DISEASES, SAME NAME

For reasons still somewhat obscure, but believed to be genetic, some people succumb to an auto-immune disease called rheumatoid arthritis. As in any auto-immune disease, the immune system, which should protect the body, instead attacks it—in this case, the joints. The synovium, or tissue that lines the inside of the joints, thickens, causing swelling and pain. Over time, cartilage erodes, reducing the space between bones in the joints and causing both instability and immobility, as well as deformity.

Others (including yours truly) develop the more common osteoarthritis.

In addition to use patterns and aging, some of us are more genetically prone to joint disarray, with osteoarthritis being the number-one offender. The Arthritis Foundation estimated in 2017 that 37% of the people in the U.S. have it. Osteoarthritis is more common in older people, though children can suffer too. And tellingly for this book, one third of people ages 18-64 have arthritis to some degree in at least some of their joints. Both aging and trauma (think: football injuries, car accidents, random falls) can lead to osteoarthritis in specific joints, and together they can conspire to make things worse. So that spill you took in your thirties might manifest as knee pain in your seventies. Massage therapists who overwork their hands often succumb to arthritis in their fingers after decades of work.

In osteoarthritis, minerals that normally circulate freely in the bloodstream throughout our bodies settle like a sediment in certain joints. The most common spots are hands, feet, and knees, but any joint can provide a proper platform.

Symptoms include pain and stiffness, especially first thing in the morning and after periods of inactivity. Movement can release both stiffness and pain, but excessive working of the joint, or movement that aggravates the inflammation, can cause more pain. Mild swelling may also appear around the joint.

Diagnosis is usually done by x-rays, which can reveal narrowing of joint space (indicating erosion of cartilage), and MRIs, which can also show the condition of soft tissue. There is no blood test for osteoarthritis, but blood work can be done to eliminate other possible conditions (rheumatoid arthritis or an infection).

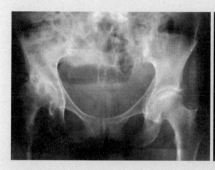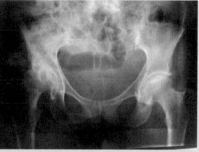

These x-rays of my hips (seen from the front), taken in July 2014, show compression of the space where the head of the femur meets its socket on the right hip, whereas the left hip shows still some space, and relatively smooth bone surfaces. Five years later, my left hip is holding up just fine!

Treatment is limited to alleviating pain with acetaminophen and nonsteroidal anti-inflammatory drugs, physical and occupational therapy, and gentle movement therapies like tai chi and yoga. Cortisone injections can provide temporary relief; joints can be surgically physically realigned, and joints can be replaced.

Here's the weird thing. Several weeks later I went back to see the rheumatologist. He projected my x-rays for both of us to see, and once more checked out my mobility on both hips. He was astounded. The x-rays showed severe arthritis, worse on the right hip, bone on bone (no cartilage left to pad the space between the top of the thigh bone and its socket). He repeated that there was no possible way I could have such extreme ROM with my degree of arthritis. But there it was!

So, he referred me to a well-respected orthopedic surgeon with a specialty in hips. (As is probably the case with many afflictions, we prospective hip patients share our contact lists, and the same handful of names pop up on everyone's lists of "the best.") He looked at my x-rays, but also noticed my extremely small bones and history of osteopenia/osteoporosis.

# HIP SURGERIES: WHAT'S THE PROBLEM? WHAT'S THE SOLUTION?

Lots of things can go wrong with your hips, and until you've had x-rays, MRIs, and other diagnostics, neither you nor your doctor can get far. Symptoms don't tell the story. That said, here's a breakdown of the most common hip surgeries:

## LABRUM TEAR REPLACEMENT

The ring of cartilage that keeps the head of the thighbone from rubbing against its socket is called the labrum. This soft tissue can get torn through accidents or progressive wear and tear. Depending on the extent of damage, surgeons can go in and stitch it back together. (By the time I got my diagnoses, I had no labrum left at all.)

## HIP RESURFACING

When there is significant arthritis (rough bone surfaces, bone spurs), you may be a candidate for hip resurfacing. Here the surgeon goes in and sands down the rough parts. This appealed to me personally, as it seemed so much less drastic than replacing the whole joint. But for reasons I don't fully understand, so far this surgery seems to work best only for large-boned young men. Being none of the three, not an option in my case.

## TOTAL HIP REPLACEMENT

As it implies, THR involves going in, sawing off the neck and head of the thighbone, and replacing them with a metal substitute custom-designed to fit your body. The implant is affixed to your body by running a long metal shaft down the thighbone toward the knee, like a sword into a sheath. The hip socket itself is replaced by a ceramic cup. The types of metal and/or ceramic vary with different manufacturers, as does the degree of mobility/stability you can expect post-op.

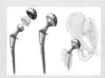 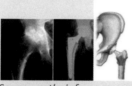 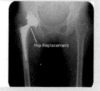

*Source: orthoinfo.aaos.org*

Historically, THR's were done by making an incision from behind, through the lateral buttocks muscles. In recent years, many surgeons have adopted an anterior approach, cutting instead through the quadriceps muscles at the front of the thigh. The latter has a quicker recovery rate. However, it's not advised for those with small and/or fragile (osteopeniac or osteoporotic) bones, as there is a higher risk of fracturing the thighbone during surgery. Given my small and brittle bones, plus the longer track record of successful outcomes, I opted for a posterior THR.

His conclusion: I was not a good candidate for a Total Hip Replacement (THR) because my brittle little twig bones could splinter during surgery, when they insert the new implant down through the thighbone like a sword into a sheath. He asked about my level of pain, which at that point was three-four-five with an occasional eight, and advised I postpone surgery as long as possible. At that point, I figured I had five to 10 years before I'd need the surgery, and that by then the technology would be that much further ahead and hopefully safer for someone of my build. Like maybe science would catch up with my great idea of creating new *padding* instead of synthetic bones—allowing them to insert a kind of silicone-breast-implant between my thighbone and its socket to ease the bone-on-bone compression and pain. So I left feeling generally good about our plan. For the moment—the brief moment, as it turns out.

That was February 2014. By April I was having pain walking more than about 15 minutes—not great in a pedestrian city like New York, where my prime means of travel to/from clients and classes is walking. By late spring I also had a pronounced limp, which was alarming my yoga students, who look to me for sound and safe practices to keep their own bodies well. I feared I'd soon be unemployed. Turning to me for guidance might seem like asking a chain smoker to help them quit cigarettes. I felt like a fraud espousing the life-enhancing gifts of yoga while feeling my own body disintegrate from the inside out.

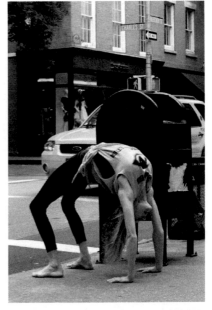

Summer came, and I made my annual migration out to the Hamptons, where I teach yoga during the resort's high season. Increasingly desperate, I decided to truly back off *all* activities that aggravated my pain. I dropped more yoga poses from my repertoire (like forward bends, hip openers/rotators, standing poses, stepping or jumping forward in the sun salutations). I tried to enjoy what was left: backbends, arm balances, inversions, and abdominal strengtheners.

So I worked the daylights out of my arms, upper body, and abs while my lower appendages withered. If this had gone on much longer I probably would have morphed into an inverted triangle like those professional weightlifters with the ginormous shoulders and tiny hips. One bright side of this reshuffling was an uptick in bone density in my forearm, which had previous dipped well below the osteoporosis line. By late summer my right leg was also noticeably thinner than the left, having atrophied from lack of use.

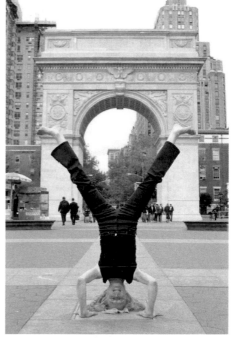

### THE FEELING UNDER THE FEELING UNDER THE FEELING . . .

So far I've focused on how scary all of this was. I was afraid for my physical wellbeing. Afraid to lose my status as a self-sufficient person who could navigate the world on two good legs. Afraid my career as a yoga teacher would come to an abrupt end, that all the years I'd put into studying, practicing, and perfecting my teaching skills would go to waste. And that I'd end up homeless. In a wheelchair.

What I haven't mentioned is how angry I was about this turn of events. I cursed God. I cursed my body for betraying me. I cursed the evil genes I'd inherited from my father's side of the family (where I traced arthritis and other forms of joint disease). Most of all I cursed myself for poor diet and lifestyle habits stretching back to my tween years, which probably exacerbated my condition. I woke up many nights to the pain and quickly transitioned to a rage that made any further sleep impossible. I'd visualize blowing up my body, my room, the house. I wanted *out*. Out of a situation that I didn't deserve and couldn't control. My best solutions always involved violence, aimed at the world, at myself, or both. I got why mass murderers shoot everyone in sight and then finish themselves off.

But under the anger was deep, deep grief. Rage inevitably sputtered out and landed me in tears. I love to move. I love to walk, run, swim, and dance.

Most of all I love yoga, which has released tension, eased anxiety, lifted dark moods, boosted my self-confidence, and taught me the value of patience, perseverance, and humility. Yoga has returned me to the person I once was as a

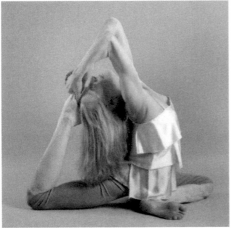

little, little kid: full of curiosity and enthusiasm, of laughter and wit. I grieved the loss of this powerful tool. I pictured returning to the high-strung, stressed-out, joyless person I was 20 years before and wondered if I'd have the will to go on. Waves of deep sadness washed over me from the beginning of my pain until my full recovery. I doubt whether more than a day or two went by between bouts of tears or morbid reflection. The helium balloon of my spirit was being dragged under water by the relentless tug of an unseen anchor. I didn't want to lose who I had become but saw no way to avoid the downward spiral.

Still, I tried all varieties of finger-in-the-dike measures. I stopped walking. Seriously. The Hamptons is a large region with no functional public

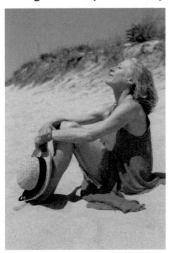

transportation, so I drove everywhere. When running (poor choice of words!) errands, I'd circle around until I found the parking space closest to my destination. I used to tease my mom for doing this ("Mom, we can walk the extra 50 feet!") but now found myself envying the folks who had those special handicapped parking permits and could snag the front spot.

I skipped events I truly enjoy, like the summer art fairs, because they involved walking over soggy fields and around airplane hangar spaces with unforgiving concrete floors. At the beach, I plunked my towel down on a direct axis between my car and the ocean, asking my friends not to walk east or west in search of less crowded areas. Walking on sand was the hardest of all, as my stabilizing muscles were shot, and the soft, slippy-slidy sand pitched all my weight into just the wrong places. Thank God the weightlessness of salt water allowed me to flipflop playfully around in the ocean. Swimming crawl stroke also worked. It was back on land that the pain shot back through me, though getting in and out also required patience and perseverance, as I was none too steady on my feet.

Despite avoiding everything I thought was troublesome, my decline between early June and mid-July was like falling off a cliff. The mantra that doctors had already told me, "You'll know when it's time [for surgery]," started to resonate. I felt like a walking structural time bomb. And I knew that my crooked gait was affecting my "good" hip, my lower back, and even my shoulders. The body is an extraordinarily complex, interconnected web, and if you pull one thread out of alignment, all the others try desperately to hold the rest together—with mixed results. I knew that as long as I relied on my body for my work as a yoga teacher, I couldn't mess with my wiring for too long without generating a chain reaction of other problems.

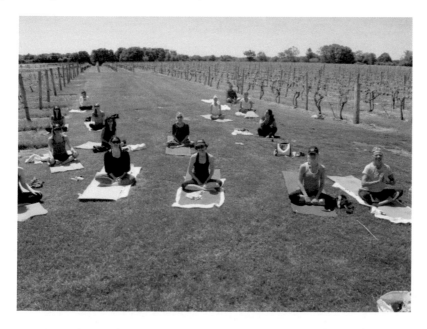

I teach outdoor classes in a vineyard during the summer, and I remember hobbling through the vines to a shade tree across the property, hiding my limp and my grimaces of pain by chatting in a chipper, lively voice with my students. It was still all-important that I hide the symptoms of my impending collapse. Looking good is everything, right?

CHAPTER THREE

# THE TIPPING POINT

*I stepped from plank to plank*
*So slow and cautiously;*
*The stars about my head I felt,*
*About my feet the sea.*

*I knew not but the next*
*Would be my final inch,—*
*This gave me that precarious gait*
*Some call experience.*

—*Emily Dickenson,*
"I stepped from plank to plank"

*Septimus Warren Smith . . . . with hazel eyes which had that look of*
*apprehension in them which makes complete strangers apprehensive too.*
*The world has raised its whip; where will it descend?*

—*Virgina Woolf, Mrs. Dalloway*

But I realized my situation had become unmanageable. I could not wait until my September return to New York City to get an updated diagnosis and hopefully some treatment. I sublet my New York apartment every summer, so getting in and out of the city via train or Hampton Jitney (bus) to see doctors posed some serious obstacles. My beloved 1994 Toyota Corolla was still hardy enough to make the rounds locally, but I simply couldn't count on her for 200-mile roundtrip odysseys. But it was time to act.

My many travels in and out of the city that summer to see doctors involved an intricate coordination of bus and train schedules, doctors' appointments, and the totally unreliable services of the New York subways and taxis—often on hot, sticky days when my spirit and my body were calling out for rest and an occasional dip in my beloved ocean. I forgot to mention above that the salt water also eased the muscles in spasm, so I usually felt pretty good for a while after. Either that, or the what most normal people consider the bone-chillingly cold water just numbed all sensation, good, bad, or indifferent throughout my body for a good few hours after each plunge!

Whenever possible I tried to do the roundtrip in one day, tallying up eight hours of travel plus moving around the city. I still remember hobbling around (I was now trying out a cane) the hard city sidewalks with the now constant searing pain sometimes bringing tears to my eyes. One endlessly generous friend, herself dealing with some pretty serious health issues, sweetly offered to let me stay in her Tribeca studio when needed. That made more than one visit possible, though the distance between "way" downtown and my Upper East Side

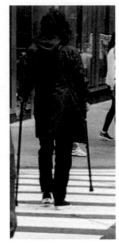

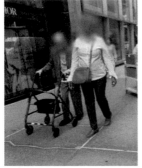

doctors induced lots of subway rides, stair-climbing, and walking. I had never thought of tiny Manhattan Island as such a huge, unnavigable tundra. Hats off to those of you who can walk! Of course, along the way, I saw many, many others limping, walking with canes, walking with walkers, maneuvering the streets and subways with less strength and stability than I still possessed.

My heart opened to them. I imagined us as the Confederacy of Cripples, soldiering along despite seemingly insurmountable obstacles. When I could, I helped others along. When we needed the subway elevator to get up to ground level, I joked and chatted with my new friends and prayed that the elevator would actually make it up and not trap us in, unnoticed and beyond help, to die a slow, pointless death. (The New York MTA is a remarkable system, but it's well over a hundred years old and grossly underfunded, so I've learned never to count on anything to actually work.) My longstanding

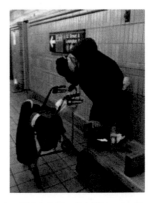

claustrophobia kicked in here. I've always been afraid of being locked in small chambers with no escape. I don't even lock the doors on public bathrooms for fear of being trapped. I'd rather have some random stranger open the door mid-pee than risk wasting away because of some malfunctioning lock. So I was delighted to have company, and the prospect of stairs, stairs, and more stairs made it worth the risk. So I often stood on a subway platform for long stretches

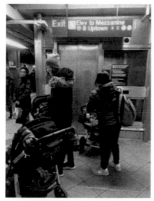

of time waiting for some other hapless invalid (or mom with a stroller, or delivery guy with a trolley) to join me, figuring at least we could play rock, paper, and scissor, charades, or Simon Says till the bitter end.

There were some bright spots. I remember climbing into the Jitney at the end of the long, traumatic day that I learned I was confirmed for surgery. I was drained and full of self-pity. Life as I knew it was coming to an end, and I could see no happy ending to this tale of woe. Those of you who have never ridden the Jitney have not sampled the bitter taste of a crowdful of entitled individuals heading to and from the Hamptons in what can only be called a bus (as much as the Jitney would have us refer to it as "a coach.") People who would like you believe that their net worth puts them in the ranks of private jets and hired helicopters but who, just for today, are slumming with the hoi polloi, forced into a $33 seat for a three-hour ride. Even the nicest people, once they mount the stairs onto the Jitney, seem to transform into edgy, snotty, and presumptuous caricatures of their better selves. They sprawl across adjacent seats. They gobble the free snacks, ask for seconds, and complain about the service. They squabble over having to pay $10 for the dog in the basket to occupy a seat next to them (claiming it's an "emotional support" dog).

Hence my surprise when I mounted at Fortieth Street and Third Avenue one summer dusk, grabbed the first available seat, and spent a few awkward minutes trying to consolidate my excess baggage into the available legroom in and around my seat. Twisting and turning every which way, I caught sight of a good-looking guy in a three-piece suit one row back smiling at me in that way . . . . To this day I cannot imagine what he found attractive in a fifty-something beanpole, wrinkled sundress thrown over the bikini I'd worn in the ocean that morning, disheveled hair, enough motley gear to qualify as a bag lady, wriggling around as gracefully as a trapped squirrel. None of this fazed him. In fact, he seemed to lean in, inviting conversation. I'm gawkish around attractive men under the best circumstances, which these were not. So I settled in, had a good cry, and prepared to suffer in silence. Still, I felt bad about snubbing him. So at some point, totally out of character, I mustered the courage to pull out a business card and scrawl on the back, "Not a good day. Still, it's lovely to see a friendly smile on the Jitney any day!" and discreetly passed it back to him. By then I guess I was actually feeling better, because I soon found myself engrossed in conversation with my seatmate, a man about my age who saw my Harvard sweatshirt, asked what class I was in, and started up. He turned out to be a neuro-psychiatrist, a new field related to my dad's profession, with lots of interesting things to say about the body-mind connection. When I happened to glance back, I noticed that Mr. Right was equally engaged in a talk with a woman who had boarded the bus later and occupied the window seat next to him. All's well that ends well, I thought. And now I don't dread the Jitney on principle, which is important, as I seem doomed to spend many an hour in that compartment of privilege.

The good news in all of this is that New York City simply has the best doctors and hospitals in the world, and I had no doubt at any point along the way that I was getting the best possible care. The bad news is, I had no options left. I had come to the end of the line. By the time I got new x-rays in July, the arthritis in my right hip had gotten dramatically worse. Every doctor I consulted agreed that I needed a total hip replacement. And as scary as that sounded, it's probably proof of the pain I was living with that I actually looked forward to surgery.

However, I faced a few logistical challenges:

- My summer subtenant in New York would not be leaving my apartment until September, so I would have no place to recuperate. East Hampton was too far away (100 miles) in case I needed emergency follow up. The house out there has three staircases I would not be able to master, and driving would be off limits for several weeks.
- I had gratefully accepted a cortisone shot in late July, and surgery is not advisable within six weeks of that. (The shot reduced my pain by about half for the first few weeks, but it was back in full flower by the time I returned to New York in early September.)
- I support myself through teaching yoga and had signed on for a full repertoire of group classes and private lessons during the busy Hamptons summer season, and I needed both to honor those commitments and keep up a revenue stream flowing for as long as possible.
- I love summer! I love throwing myself in the ocean several times a day. I love my home in East Hampton, my four-poster bed that I take to like a puppy to its basket. I love quiet nights and dark skies. I did not want to give up one day of all that, pain or no pain.

September is always a funny transition month, with summer routines coming to an end, kids going back to school, and Jewish holidays, so I figured I would be less missed during that month. We scheduled the surgery for September 11, a date none of us will forget, and I began the long, tedious, sobering path of preparing for the big day.

## IF AND WHEN . . . WOULD SOMEONE PLEASE CALL A DOCTOR?

As I made my preliminary rounds of doctor consults, I would ask each specialist whether I should have the surgery. The universal answer? "You'll know when it's time." By which, I now know, they meant the point at which chronic pain escalates into frequent agony during simple daily movements like walking a city block.

That's exactly when I went under the knife—or pneumatic drill, as I now understand it was. In my informal canvassing of other THR candidates, I've seen people whom I personally believe are living with unacceptable limitations and should have had the operation years

## DON'T TRY THIS AT HOME-UNLESS YOU HAVE TO

I heard that when *Eat, Pray, Love* became an international bestseller, it propelled legions of women to strike out on their own worldwide odysseys of self-discovery (and many I would guess with high hopes of landing a prince like Elizabeth Gilbert's at the end). Weirder still is the phenomenon of women catapulted off their couches into wilderness treks inspired by Cheryl Strayed's *Wild,* an account of her gutsy if ill-conceived plan to hike the 1,000-mile Pacific Crest Trail solo, with no experience of either hiking or camping.

While I intend for this book to inspire each of you to rise to your highest, *please* understand that by no means am I advocating total hip replacements for all! Even if you are a likely candidate for same, major surgery deserves careful forethought. Read the fine print. Pay attention to potential side effects—like death—of the surgery itself and long-term limitations (I'm never supposed to run again; many hip replacements wear out and have to be replaced by replacements; implants are magnets for infections, etc.). You're not, in other words, buying an open-ended boarding pass. You're agreeing to incorporate a significant piece of inanimate hardware into your body for life. And while the state of the art is pretty high, no one can guarantee that these implants are trouble-free.

ago. I also occasionally come across people who opt for surgery prophylactically, which strikes me as medical overkill. Opinions aside, here are the pros and cons of waiting, jumping the gun, or acting just in the knick:

<u>CALLING ALL PROCRASTINATORS</u>

What you'll gain:

- Surgical technologies get better every day. The longer you wait, the better the techniques available and the more experience the physicians will have with the newer methods. For example, the "anterior" approach to THR was relatively new when I chose the more traditional "posterior" approach. I gambled on the tried and true over the newest inspiration, but happily in this case I've heard of successes with both methods, at least in the short run.
- You can schedule the time required for surgery and post-op physical therapy for a time that's as convenient as possible for you. You can minimize the temporary limitations in your ability to do things like drive a car, climb in and out of the bathtub, or take a dip in the ocean.

What you'll lose:

- Countless nights of good sleep, as hip pain can often be worst at night, gradually eroding the quality of your daylight hours and your overall health.
- The ability to do some things you used to love, like taking long walks, gardening, doing a full-spectrum yoga class, etc.
- You're not getting any younger! Youthful bodies recover from major surgeries faster and more reliably. Increasingly brittle bones (a hallmark of aging) also put you at risk of fracture as the surgeon saws through your femur bone to insert the implant.

<u>EAGER BEAVERS BEWARE</u>

What you'll gain:

- I've heard people say they want to get it over with before things get really bad. This logic undoubtedly applies to some medical procedures, like removing cancerous or precancerous tissues and installing potentially life-saving pacemakers. Apparently it's advised for rotator-cuff tears in the shoulder joint, where the longer you wait, the harder it

39

is to stitch things back together. With THR, going in early might spare you some months of pain and restore good sleep as mentioned above, though none of the doctors I consulted suggested that earlier was better.

What you'll lose:

- As mentioned above, surgical technologies are advancing at a rapid clip, especially for such universally common procedures as hip replacements. The longer you wait, the better the techniques employed, the surgeon's skills, and the implants installed.
- You may never need the surgery at all. While x-rays showed pretty severe arthritis in both of my hips, I'm five years past my first THR and my second hip is 100% asymptomatic. With a bit of luck, it might see me through until the end!

### TIMING IS EVERYTHING (WAITING TILL YOU KNOW IT'S TIME)

What you'll gain:

- The satisfaction of knowing you'll receive the most up-to-date treatment available.
- The cold comfort (certainty) that you had no other options—no buyer's remorse, no wouldha-couldha-shouldha.

What you'll lose:

- Quality of life for the last excruciating weeks or months between when you know it's time and when you are able to schedule a surgery with a doctor you trust.
- The patience to take your time, hem and haw over options, do extra research, get second, third, and fourth opinions.
- The leisure to choose a "good" time to have the surgery (during summer or winter, during a lull in your work life or a time you foresee buckling down to a lot of sedentary work anyway, etc.).

Those are the broad strokes as I see 'em. Of course it's up to you, dear reader, to map out your own path. I'm not a doctor, an expert, a guru, or a self-help motivator.

I also have to come clean about how I see what led me, the 55-year-old acrobat, to the OR for a total hip replacement. This is crucial reading, my friends, because I'm afraid many of my yoga students, acquaintances, and colleagues see me as some kind of invincible creature who has defied the laws of both gravity (one-arm handstands) and aging (I can do stuff many 14 year olds will never master). You may also assume that:

- I adhere to some rigorously pure "yogi" diet. Hardly. I often pick up an antibiotic-laden rotisserie chicken from the local grocery store and eat it for five days straight. Oh, and I have that girl thing about frozen yogurt.
- I never smoke (true).
- I never drink (well, not anymore).
- I'm free of prescription drugs (nope! I'm as chemically dependent on doctor prescribed pharmaceuticals as the next American).

Food and drugs aside, you may think that as a yoga teacher, I devote a good portion of each day/week to practicing yoga. While I probably lead the pack here, having the luxury of no kids and no full-time job, it's true that I don't practice *every day*, and I'm more likely to over- than under-do it. Meaning I'll practice strenuously even when I'm tired, sick, or injured, thus defeating the purpose.

Perhaps you also assume that I meditate daily. Not true. Aside from my yoga practice, walking, and swimming (meditation in motion) and the mantra repetition I do during prolonged periods of insomnia, I simply cannot or will not sit on cushion, on the floor, and do "nothing" unless I am under the supervision of a teacher/class/group/peer-pressure setting. Thus I consciously or unconsciously avoid what many medical practitioners, East and West, concur is the most potent route to healing. Master meditation teacher Sylvia Boorstein wrote a book called *Don't Just Do Something, Sit There!* Love the title, but sadly, I'd rather do just about *anything* than sit still and alone with my crazy brain.

Truth is, I'm erratic with my diet, my yoga practice, and just about everything else in my life. And I pay the price. Chalk it up to undiagnosed (but painfully obvious) Attention Deficit Disorder, but I'm as inconsistent in my friendships and work habits as in my healthcare regime. This book could have been finished months ago if I knew how to stick to a schedule. Instead, I feel like I'm constantly juggling too many balls and dropping most of them most of the time.

So, despite my years of yoga and spiritual *intentions*, I'm not at all sure that I'm really any further along the path than most of you. I do run across what I call "natural yogis," people who seem to have gotten it right the first time around. For me, it's more like a game of catch up. Consider me damaged goods, and all of my spiritual and physical practices as remedial efforts to return me to the healthy body God gave me way back when. So I guess I am an average bear after all. Which is painful to admit for someone who, from early childhood, parents and teachers and just about everyone else saw as exceptional. Or maybe I'm just more a creature of extremes: all on, incredibly focused and yes, talented, at the things I do *when* I do them, disciplined to the point of rigidity when I'm "in control," then a hopeless scattershot disaster when on free range.

So heading into major surgery, I gave myself a 50/50 chance of a successful outcome.

CHAPTER FOUR

# I'M NOT JUST TALKING ABOUT HIPS!

*About suffering they were never wrong,*
*The old Masters: how well they understood*
*Its human position: how it takes place*
*While someone else is eating or opening a window or just walking dully*
*along.*

—W.H. Auden, "Musee des Beaux-Arts"

*One of mankind's greatest misunderstandings is that there is more than*
*one of us.*

—Albert Einstein

Before we move on, I also want to be clear that this book is *not* just about...

- Hips, healthy or unhealthy.
- Joints, healthy or not.
- Bodies in any way, shape, form or misformation.
- Yoga.
- Yoga's effects, good and not so good, on the body.

I'm well aware that not everyone will face a hip problem (thank God!) and that many readers may never come within down-dog distance of a yoga mat (or a yoga studio). I've already cultivated a growing network of hip peers. We support and inform each other through asking for help from those who have had hip surgeries (or are contemplating the same). And especially those who have had joint problems very likely associated with yoga and other forms of physical exercise that require extreme range of motion. I hope they'll all enjoy this read, identify with much of what I've been through, and share it with other fellow travelers. But since that network is already alive and thriving, I didn't feel I needed to write a book for them—or at least not *just* for them.

The real point of this book is to inspire anyone facing one of life's curveballs—and everyone does. I'm focused here on the paradox of an advanced yogi and yoga teacher trainer reduced to a cripple, with all of the personal anguish and public shame that brought on. But everybody goes through something—injuries, illnesses, breakups, layoffs, and losses of every stripe. If I learned anything from this journey, and it may sound cliché, often what seems like the worst thing that could possibly happen turns out to be the best. I'm fully aware that those words may sound hollow to anyone currently in the throes of unbearable pain, deep mourning, or paralyzing fear. I also know that it doesn't take something as catastrophic as major surgery to reduce me to any of those states. The darndest little things can throw me off beam in a heartbeat.

And that's still not okay with me. I guess I've never accepted that life is no bowl of cherries, that each day cannot be one blissful moment followed by another in a pink cloud of euphoria. I've tried desperately to achieve this through any means available. I've thrown myself into myriad pursuits—playing the piano, swimming crazy amounts of miles up and down endless pools, sailing, tennis, singing, making art, writing—that completely absorb me and push my worries to the periphery. Until I can't master a given piece on the piano, an artwork goes south, or I hit writer's block, at which point I plunge back into the darkness. I've tried compulsive socializing to distract me. When people have let me down (or proved more trouble than they're worth!), I've put myself in the isolation tank—which inevitably leads to a monstrous expansion of pain, grief, or fear. And when all reasonably healthy options have failed, I've turned to alcohol and drugs (prescription and the other kind) to allow me to zone out. And we all know where that leads.

So, those of you with happy hips, what can you get out of this book? Hopefully my hard-won conviction that you can move through your darkest hours and come out shining. Here are a few of mine:

I'm by nature optimistic and cheery, but I'd be lying if I said that there weren't some pretty dark moments along the way into and out of my surgery. I was usually able to make light of these—or at least see the light ahead—but they deserve mention along with the stuff that went so well. So here are some glimpses of the shadow side:

WALK DON'T RUN, AND FORGET ABOUT THE STAIRS!

*You're in pretty good shape for the shape you're in.*

*—Dr. Seuss*

At the hospital and in doctors' offices, they're always asking you to rate your pain on at scale of 1 to 10. At best, in the early days, there were still some zones of every day or night when I was at 0. At worst, I was creeping up to about 8, and unfortunately walking and climbing stairs—pretty crucial to survival anywhere, but especially in pedestrian NYC—were the worst.

45

Alas, by June 1, the pain was pretty much constant. Fortunately, by then I was set up in East Hampton for the summer, so I could pretty much avoid walking (car culture with everything spread out). But I couldn't avoid the stairs to my bedroom, so I invented Climbing Dog—basically like Downward Facing Dog, done climbing up the stairs on two hands and two feet. If I was feeling patient (or was in a public place where Climbing Dog would attract attention and concern), I would walk up the stairs always leading with the "good" leg and following with the bad one. Good leg,

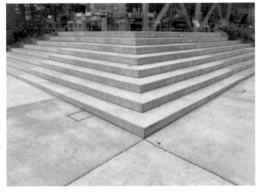

bad leg. Good leg, bad leg. Painfully slow. My favorite staircase was the one to my basement, because it has railings on both sides, and I could hoist myself up rock-climber style by using my arms instead of my legs. I remember about that time reading a fitness article by pop-doctor Andrew Weill, who recommended walking 20 minutes a day, and finished by saying *anyone* can walk!" Not so, and I now see how such broad statements can inadvertently discourage the rest of us.

ABOUT THAT BASEMENT

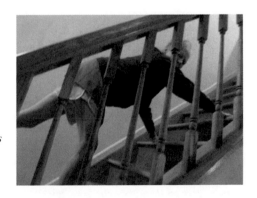

*Oh, the thinks you can think!*

*—Dr. Seuss*

I have either an incredibly high metabolism or an innate sensitivity to heat, or both. I am basically always too hot, and could easily be put to better use as a human generator or space heater. I open windows and doors in midwinter, sleep with a fan on high-speed aimed right at my bed *and* air-conditioning in the summer, and can be seen strolling about in tank shirts and shorts when others are bundled head to toe.

To conserve on our A/C bills, as well as to limit my exposure to the summer sun that streams through my East Hampton greenhouse-like living/dining area, I set up a desk in the basement, where the temperature hovers around 60 degrees. I spent long hours in my summer cave, responding to emails, negotiating overseas teaching, making art, working out. While I was definitely more comfortable down there, it is absolutely true that dark environments lead to dark thoughts. As my hip pain worsened and it looked like surgery was my only recourse, it was in my little basement cell that I had to do things that wouldn't be fun anywhere, including:

- Phone calls and emails with friends for whom THR had not gone well
- Diving into the ever-shifting web of doctors and insurance plans, sorting out my options and assessing the dizzying costs.
- Convincing my dad that I was not a princess demanding the priciest care out there but a thoughtful, thrifty person scared shitless about how this was all going to hit my bottom line (in fact, the time and money sunk into this project dragged me well down below that line, and I'm still struggling to recoup my losses).
- Revising my will, living will, and power of attorney. Thank God I had created those documents years ago while enjoying good health, as I doubt I would have been so clear about the insights and intentions contained therein (who does what, who gets what, how to deal with an incapacitated Lois). I love my family members and the organizations I plan to leave my legacy. But still, having to review all of this with the prospect of leaving *myself* was *not* fun.

I've never understood moderation, and it's kind of appropriate that I went from having *never* had surgery (just a few minor procedures), to having a pretty major, invasive, bone slicing and rearranging, metal-and-ceramic implanting surgery. (As my physical therapist noted, if you want to see how a Total Hip Replacement actually goes down, there are YouTube videos that capture the whole process. I was curious, until he added that it was like a chain saw or power drill going through concrete, "This Old House" on this old body is how he summed it up. I decided to pass.)

So, medically speaking, I soared from zero to 60 in one dramatic leap. Yet oddly, despite the enormity of what I was about to undergo, I found myself actually looking forward to The Day. And, being pretty much in perpetual motion (always on trains or planes, walking everywhere, doing hours of yoga and Physique 57 every day—once took three barre classes in one day!), I found myself actually looking forward to having a legitimate excuse to not go *anywhere* or even *move*. I piled up a stash of good books, updated my Netflix queue, and alerted the staff in my apartment building that I was expecting to be immobilized for some time.

Exercising my increasingly disabled body meant eliminating jumping (as in sun salutes), any kind of hip flexion (folding forward), internal and external rotation of my right leg, and anything standing. So I worked the daylights out of my arms, upper body, and abs while my lower appendages withered. If this had gone on much longer I probably would have morphed into an inverted triangle like those professional weightlifters with the ginormous shoulders and tiny hips. One bright side of this reshuffling was an uptick in bone density in my forearm, which had previous dipped well below the osteoporosis line.

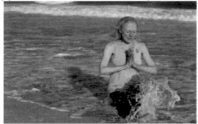

I could swim, but walking on the sand down to the water was excruciating. A friend had given me a gorgeous turquoise wetsuit so that I could stay in the frigid water longer, but getting in and out of the suit required some pretty painful gyrations. I had promised a fashion designer photos of myself in her newest line of yoga clothes. Not being sure I'd ever be doing yoga again after The Day, I rushed to get some videos and photos shot in July. My assistant Say and I had to work around all the things I *couldn't* do (like standing, rotating my legs in or out, forward bending, binding, and most twists). Even so, I had tears of pain in my eyes as I struggled to hold the poses long enough for her to get good shots.

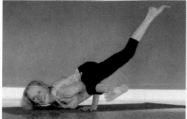 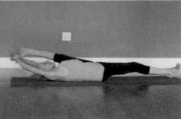

However, I'm glad we made the effort, as I sensed my doctors had no idea of what I considered normal physical activity. Guessing that the description "yoga teacher" implied someone who sat cross-legged in meditation for hours on end, I dropped that moniker and started calling myself an acrobat. This turned out to be quite shrewd, as it got my doctors' attention and clarified my expectations to both the surgeon and my post-op physical therapist. Basically I wanted to still be able to put my foot behind my head when reached 100 years old. Well, they did ask!

Perhaps the really low point was my return to New York City in the fall of 2014—exactly three days before my surgery. I had only a few things to accomplish, stuff that would have been easy for anyone with two functioning legs. I was visibly limping. One of my favorite doormen, who knows I spend my summers out near the ocean, saw me limping and innocently joked, "Waves too big?" I tried to laugh but with the pain at that point, all I could do was to muster a grimace and pick up my mail before hopping the elevator to my fourth-floor apartment.

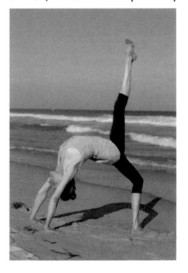

The next challenge was visiting my lawyer's office near Grand Central Station to sign my revised will, living will, and power of attorney. I bravely tackled the subways (ouch, stairs and more stairs!) to his office, only to discover he had moved to the East Thirties. Somehow I snagged a taxi to his new office, but I arrived 45 minutes late, with tears of pain streaming down my cheeks.

We got the papers signed, but exiting his office at rush hour, with rain coming down, I hailed taxis in vain for a good half hour. Finally I gave up and tried to find the nearest subway. I limped along in the rain for blocks and blocks, only to find a subway that still deposited me even more blocks from home.

The next day Say came over to help me rearrange my apartment so that everything I needed to reach would be at hip height or higher. (I had been told that post-op I would not be able to bend more than 90 degrees forward.)

We set up a spare card table with all of my books, papers, and laptop, and a second table for dining. We unfolded my futon couch (knee high) and inflated an Aerobed to stack on top of it, raising my bed so high I would have to stand on a chair to get in or out of it. We made sure I had food on the top shelf of the fridge. We installed a raised toilet seat with handles (a last-minute purchase from Amazon that proved the most worthwhile investment of all). I

49

passed on the bathtub supports, unclear how to install them and assuming I would just shower my way through or live in filth for awhile since I didn't foresee any socializing on the horizon.

As we were winding down in the late afternoon, I decided to walk one short block east to pick up a rotisserie chicken at Gourmet Garage, and then a short block west to get a massage (needless to say my body was clenched up like a vise and I desperately craved some release). Alas, I made it to the Garage and picked up my chicken. But that short walk had been so painful that I sat down on the bench in front of the store and cried. Forget about walking the 100 yards past my place to the massage. It was dawning on me that if the hip surgery didn't work, I was not going to be able to live in Manhattan. Unless I took to a wheelchair.

CHAPTER FIVE

**THE DAY**

"No worst, there is none. Pitched past pitch of grief,
More pangs will, schooled at forepangs, wilder wring."

—*Gerald Manley Hopkins*

*Weather forecast for tonight: dark. Continued dark overnight, with widely
scattered light by morning.*

—*George Carlin*

So by now you have a pretty good idea of where I was, mentally and physically, by the time The Day, September 11, 2014, the date of my actual surgery, arrived.

Of course most New Yorkers, if they were marking that day in any way, were probably recalling the horrific events of September 11, 2001. And it did provide some freedom from the bondage of self to realize what small fry my day held compared with what others had suffered 13 years before—lives ended or permanently mangled by injury and grief. How many lives had been cut short or irrevocably altered? A cityscape permanently changed, along with the bravura that created it.

But back to my little world. Having only landed in New York City two days before, I was experiencing the annual trauma of adjusting to city noise, crowds, and heat after summer out by the sea. My pre-op protocol had also required that for the past week I go cold turkey on all of the herbs, supplements, and prescription drugs that keep me functioning as normally as possible. I was weak, disoriented, and deprived of my usual chemical fortifications. I guess I should also have been scared, but thankfully my trust in my surgeon, my hospital, and the promise of relief from unbearable pain (and, as with all major looming events, the desire to just get it over with) actually made me eager to wheel into the OR.

A few notes here about being single/no kids in New York City or just about anywhere else in our fine Land of the Free. The law (reasonably) requires that anyone going in for any hospital procedure (and this includes routine outpatient events like colonoscopies) be accompanied by another, non-medicated adult. I'd been through this drill a few times before, so I knew it was a deal-breaker. I enlisted one absolutely 100% reliable friend to meet me at my apartment in the *lower west* West Village and car service up to the Hospital for

Special Surgery at Manhattan's farthest corner—the Upper *far upper* East Side. As a backup, I enlisted Say to meet us in the waiting room.

Having spent my share of hours in the now-defunct (and greatly missed) Saint Vincent's emergency room after the bike accident, a broken finger, a gashed hand, a rogue contact lens, and other assorted mishaps, as well as waiting waiting waiting in doctors' offices, I assumed that the three of us would be there till . . . whenever.

To my surprise, the well-oiled wheels of HSS kept everything rolling along on schedule. I was admitted, with one friend, into the pre-op chamber where you wait for your turn under the knife.

Here life tossed up an unexpected gift. One of my students, who had been through way more and way worse than I in the preceding year, asked her son-in-law to pop in on me pre-op and make sure I was being well handled. Turns out he works for the hospital and skipped away from his usual duties to wish me well. Note to readers: it's been my experience that the people who happen to surround us in our highest highs and lowest lows are rarely those (or exclusively those) we rank as our inner circle.

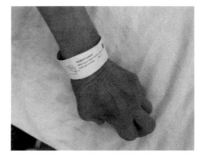

It was only in the last few minutes, with my good friend by my bedside, that my courage finally caved. I was scared. Nope, I was terrified. If this didn't work, I'd be a lifetime invalid without the financial, familial, or social resources to see it through. I saw myself, once the active, acrobatic, self-sustaining individual, passing the rest of my days in a "rest" home, at best spinning around in a wheel chair, at worst, in permanent bed rest. And given the marginal state of my finances, the open question of who would bankroll such a life lurked over the whole dismal scenario.

About that time, the anesthesiologist arrived to remind me I'd be going under and possibly might not resurface. Oh joy, here we go! Needless to say, I was in tears by the time they arrived to wheel me into the OR. As I was "going under," I still remember an angel of a nurse who took one look at me, declared, "Why are you crying? It's a party in there, a party for you!" All I remember before I blacked out was the smiling faces of the OR team and Frank Sinatra playing the background. Not my choice of relaxing soundtrack, but at that point, I was willing to surrender my will, my tastes, my energy, and my personality to anyone who had a clue what to do with my hip.

Being really, really good at a handful of things and hopelessly inadequate in everything else, I'm actually pretty good at surrendering. Not sure where I got this gift. The person I most consistently resemble on this planet is my dad, who never surrenders anything. Years ago he went into the hospital for a routine gallbladder operation that didn't go so well. The staff decided he should remain in the hospital under observation for another five days. A doctor himself, dear old Dad reached down to the foot of his bed, where his chart was stashed in a folder. He read through the chart, decided he was fine, and checked himself out of the hospital without so much as consulting another physician. Imagine the nurses' surprise when the entered his room to find his bed empty!

I, on the other hand, would come to enjoy HSS's cheerful staff, the views of the East River from almost every waiting room and hospital bed, having a staff of dozens of nurses, physician's assistants, doctors, specialists, nurse's aides, and administrators looking after me so much that the prospect of ever returning home to my solitary life was growing less and less appealing.

My surgery apparently went splendidly (I was so doped up I missed the whole event). I remember my surgeon coming down to the recovery room and high-fiving me that all was well, and my assistant coming by to say she was on her way home.

All *was* well! Until it wasn't. Most patients spend two to three hours in the recovery room before being transported up to a bed for the night. I've even heard of a couple of THR patients who were sent home the day or their surgery. I, alas, faced a couple of major obstacles:

- Every hour, a physical therapist (PT) or physician's assistant (PA) would come by and ask me to wiggle my (right foot/surgery side) toes. Nothing doing. As far as I was concerned, the leg was "dead." Hate to use that word, but when there's no sensation/no movement, better words fail!
- In the so-called "recovery room," while I was waiting/hoping for my leg to wake up, I had the gift of a true wrench in the bed next to me. For a good three hours straight she moaned, whined, complained, demanded extra care. Every moment I tried to drift off into post-op sleep, she was there to keep me awake, alive, enervated. Even the nurses started ignoring her incessant demands.

Afternoon drifted into evening. 2:00pm, 4:30, 6:30, 9:00. My difficult neighbor was transferred upstairs, only to be replaced by an equally squawky individual.

By about 10:00pm everyone had concurred that something was amiss with me and my leg. Being ever-inquisitive, I gleaned from whoever drifted by that sometimes hip replacements can "displace" the sciatic nerve—the nerve that activate your whole leg from your hip down to your toes. Usually, the damage is temporary, but again, no guarantees. A friend had had a THR in Mexico during which they accidentally severed the sciatic nerve, leading to a follow-up surgery and months of pain. What if mine never woke up? Just when I thought I was out of the woods, things were looking pretty grim.

## FLASHLIGHTS FOR THE DARK
## NIGHTS OF THE SOUL

We all get hit with them. Catastrophic events that topple expectations and warp our carefully crafted visions of where we are going. The all-too-human response? Panic, denial, anger, outrage, terror, grief—any or all of the above, often whipped into an unpalatable brew that poisons our minds and hearts.

While my life has been blessedly free of the worst examples of such calamities, I've suffered enough to acquire a few tools. Nothing that's guaranteed to make the pain go away, but small things to keep your thoughts moving in the right direction

# THE FOUR STAGES OF TRAUMA

I didn't make this one up, but it's the best description I know of what to expect:

    1. DENIAL: Nope, it didn't happen. It's not happening. It's not gonna happen. Etc., etc. Flying in the face of evidence and reason, denial is nonetheless a truly life-preserving response. Kinda like when your physical body goes into shock cuz it just can't process extreme trauma, or when you heart shuts down (goes numb) rather than feeling loss, insult, or injury. We can fly along on the wings of desire, floating above just about any grim reality, for astonishingly long periods of time. In doubt? Check out Joan Dideon's *The Year of Magical Thinking*, in which a first-class intellect continues to doubt that her husband has actually died, well beyond the actual event.

    2. ANGER: When denial crumbles under irrefutable reality, we rebel. We admit things have gone wrong, horribly wrong. And we're furious. Why me? Why now? Why am I being punished? What about them? Or, in its most humble form: Why did I bring this down on myself? Anger is a powerful source of energy, but one that's just about impossible to channel in any positive direction. Its outward vector damages others; turned inward, we self-destruct. Think of mass shooters who gun down perfect strangers then shoot themselves. I've found the only safe way to deal with anger is to wait it out while praying for the willingness not to act on it. Watching action movies (cars blowing up, buildings toppling, natural and manmade destruction), listening to garage-band noise music, playing sadistic video games, or just visualizing doing violent things can all let off steam.

    3. ACCEPTANCE: As the sound and the fury abate, at least for brief spells, a kind of quiet surrender descends. We adjust to what's happening, seeing it without fighting it. But acceptance does not mean resignation. The latter leads to complacency, self-pity, passivity, paralysis. The former paves the way for action, enabling us to see what is and envision what we can do about it.

4. ACTION: Stage Four, where we finally get up and do whatever we can: visit doctors, find a therapist, call a lawyer, send out a few resumes, jump back into the stream of life. Participate in our healing, our recovery, our return to being solid, self-supporting citizens.

In my humble experience, you can't skip over any of these steps and still get where you want to go. That said, they don't usually manifest in a predictable linear progression either. Expect a tortuous path with plenty of backslides and reversals, at least a few eddies (miring in the quicksand is how it usually feels to me), and an occasional flying leap forward. While it's a tough suggestion, being where you are is more fruitful than bemoaning the past or dreading the future.

## FINGERS IN THE DIKE

Once you're realized you're in a pickle, with limited options, your mind may start to implode, sucking you into the black hole of self-pity. Here are a few tools that can lead you back to the light.

1. Gratitude lists: When self-pity descends, make a list (written is best but mental will do) of three, five, or ten things in your life just as it is today for which you are truly grateful. Can be as simple as the taste of your morning coffee or a ray of sun that bends around a building and beams down on your face. Or a quiet neighbor in the next bed over.

2. Helping others: Doesn't have to be showing up at soup kitchen. Can be little stuff like helping an older person up the subway stairs or putting a hand of sympathy on the shoulder of a grieving friend.

3. Helping others anonymously: Doing random acts of kindness for people who will never know *you* did them, thus bypassing the ego's incessant need for praise while reminding us that our contributions are usually pretty damn small—stuff we should be doing all the time without expecting kudos.

4. Plugging back into your web: Hopefully by now I've stressed the importance of fellow travelers. They're the folks we need most when we're down and out. And letting them help us makes them feel better too!

5. Change the channel: I'm so glad my days are full with work, with people, with getting out of the house and moving around the world. The best way out of a funk is to stop dwelling on it by turning your attention to something—anything!—else.

6. Take a walk. Preferably with your dog, who you are then serving. But even the dogless among us benefit from movement, and moving around in the outer world, especially the natural world, is a foolproof way to take the focus off our own suffering.

As I lay there, I faced the prospect that perhaps I would never walk again. Or do yoga. Or swim in the ocean. Or . . . the picture grew darker and darker. Until one of life's little miracles occurred. Chalk it up to 20 years of yoga and an equal number of years of 12-step recovery, plus a hearty dose of Tantric philosophy that constantly reminds us that life is a gift (not a penance), but something shifted inside that I could never have consciously directed. I said, "Yes!" Yes to being a cripple, yes to a life in a wheelchair, yes to whatever was left. I realized that if I couldn't use my body, I could still use my mind, my eyes, my ears. I could write, I could make art, I could connect to the world in so many other ways. At the deepest level, I realized that I would be fine.

I couldn't have forced that feeling to surface. No amount of affirmations or prayers could have led me there. I realized that I had simply, and profoundly, become a different person than the girl who always, desperately needed everything to be *perfect*. Who felt she was just barely getting by using *all* of her God-given abilities. I now carry the thought that I will *always* be fine with me consciously, daily. I've given up (for the most part), the need to write life's script—which never worked anyway.

Looking back on the past few years, I realized I'd already been through some pretty scary stuff:

- About two years before my surgery, my long-term yoga teacher got exposed in a scandal that sent my professional community and identity tumbling into the dust. In addition to the weird disillusionment with his character (like many in our yoga community, I had had no idea of the nefarious doings he'd been up to for quite some time), I faced a career crisis. I severed my affiliation with that yoga "brand," and in the process lost half my students, a good part of my position as a prominent teacher on the yoga "stage," and more than half of my income.
- About the same time, a yoga teacher I'd worked for and alongside for 20 years fired me for various shortcomings that seemed small to me but huge to him. Another revenue stream ended abruptly. But more importantly, I found myself cut off from the many students and friends I had cultivated while teaching at his studio those many long years. I was isolated, lonely, depressed. Yet careful not to speak poorly and publicly of my colleague's judgment, I was unable to convey to my students why I was no longer on the schedule; I crawled away in silence to keep my side of the street clean.
- A year later my best friend and confidante betrayed me. Not for the first time, it turns out, but the breach of trust left me not only lonely but questioning my judge of character.

I can't honestly say that I dealt with these events gracefully or easily. My health suffered. My self-esteem suffered. I had to borrow money from my aging parents just to meet my monthly expenses. I wobbled forward on shaky legs, like a young fawn learning how to walk without a mother to guide her. The littlest stuff threw me off-balance. My anxiety soared. I spent less time with people and more time trying to brood my way out of my fear and my misery. I remember at the time of the yoga scandal, my dad predicted it would take me a couple of years to get back on my feet, financially and professionally. We're well into year four. While I can honestly say that my teaching and knowledge have improved exponentially, as has my confidence in what I do, maintaining my professional position in this ever-shifting world remains a daily challenge.

Unbeknownst to me, my PA called my surgeon to fill him in on what was going down. It was now close to midnight, and despite the dopey meds, I was wide awake, all systems firing.

Somehow, in a hospital full of now occupied beds, they found a room where I could pass the night and hopefully get some rest. Away from fluorescent lights, away from disturbing neighbors, I was done. Except of course I couldn't sleep—who could, facing such a life-changing predicament? This was truly my dark night of the soul.

But I must have finally drifted off, because I still remember waking up at dawn, just as the sun was starting to stream through my window. I wiggled my toes, left and right. Woohoo! I could finally feel a little something, just a tingling but at least *something,* on the right. About 10 minutes later my doctor entered my room. Turns out he had offered to spend the night in the hospital with me, but my PA had wisely pointed out that there was really nothing he could do but wait it out with the rest of us.

Within the next hour and a half, my toes, then my foot, then my leg gradually woke up. It turned out that it was not the surgery but the post-op "block" (painkillers) that had done the damage. I am small, and I have very thin legs without much muscle mass. Apparently they gave me too much post-op medication. Having filled up my muscles, the extra meds migrated into my sciatic nerve, temporarily numbing the nerve.

I was going to walk again! I might even be able to do yoga—or swim in the ocean, or dance, or drive a car. My cup runneth over! Praise the Lord.

CHAPTER SIX

**THE DAY AFTER**

So there I was, sprung back to my normal, goal-oriented, ambitious self. Doing my best to be patient, I gobbled down my breakfast (true to form, HSS provided a groaning board of scrambled egg wrap, oatmeal, fruit salad, and tea, with a Gerbera daisy laid sweetly across the whole affair). And started planning my exit strategy.

The physical therapist appeared mid-morning. I'd been told not to expect to be "pampered" post-op. The new, improved method is to force patients up and out of bed for rigorous activity within hours of surgery. Of course, given my temporarily "dead" leg, I was granted a grace period untill the next morning. Given my usual—okay, unusual—level of physical activity, I was prepped for Tough Love.

That's not exactly how it went down. Basically, the PT edged me gingerly up to a seated position, pivoted me around so my legs hung over the side of the bed, and propped me up on a walker so I could use my arms instead of my legs for support. We sallied out into the hallway, and paced up and down twice. Given that the hall might have been 100 feet long, I was just warming up when the PT guided me back to bed. Hello!

Of course I did notice while we trundled up and down that I was by far the youngest person on my ward. Most patients were in their late 70s to 90s, frail in every sense of the word and obviously challenged by the stroll down Hallway Lane. But I was done. I was, I thought, up and ready to tackle Manhattan.

My surgeon had said that morning that I could leave whenever I felt I was ready. Fortified by breakfast and cocky about my ambulatory skills, I checked myself out. Then around noon, a nurse came around and asked if I was feeling any pain. Yup. Without further discussion she IV'd another dose of Oxycodone. Before I knew what hit me, I was spacey, nauseous, and incoherent. The prospect of navigating my way from the Upper East Side to the West Village during Friday evening rush hour seemed less plausible. My parents and siblings, far from New York City, were also encouraging me to stay put for another night.

I'm still not sure why I was so driven to get home, as I had no husband or kids awaiting my return, no cats to feed, no work to do. I guess the deal-breaker was that the meds made me feel worse (tired but unable to sleep), added to the fact that as long as you stay in a hospital, they are required to wake you up every four hours to check your "vitals." So in essence I wasn't getting the rest I desperately needed to heal.

So, spacey, nauseous, and exhausted, I stayed at HSS Friday night. The hospital continued to outdo itself in meal prep. Two hours before dinner, a nutritionist came in to take my order! I was offered a choice of entrees, sides, etc. from a detailed printed menu. And told I could make a special request if none of the numerous offerings appealed to me. I remember ordering grilled salmon and veggies, so looking forward to a meal as the highlight of my day, only to find myself too nauseated to eat a bite.

I spent the rest of that night listening to my roommate, recipient of some kind of back surgery, toss, turn, moan, and demand more medication.

By Saturday morning, I'd had enough. I requested a release and lined up my trusty friend to allow us to exit ASAP. Alas, it turns out, Saturday is not a high-functioning day for Manhattan hospitals. Doctors, nurses, and hospital staff are people too, and as chaotic as their work lives may sometimes be, they apparently share the common folk's healthy respect for weekends.

We waited, and we waited, and we waited. Finally, about three hours after schedule, a young male assistant nurse came in to dress me. I still find it weird, in these days of widespread alarm over sexual harassment/innuendos, that this is the one hospital employee who saw me buck naked. Not that I have anything to hide, but as a 50+ woman it's still a little uncomfortable to be stripped and then dressed by a 20-something hulk.

As my friend and I gathered my stuff together to head home, the hospital bestowed me with a cane and a walker. I had been advised that when using a walker, it's really important to have a basket attached to carry whatever you need from place to place, since both hands are steering the walker. So my friend and I spent most of the long ride home dialing surgical supply stores, then Bed Bath and Beyond, and finally bicycle stores and hardware stores, hoping to outfit my walker with a suitable basket.  No one could promise that their baskets would fit. Finally, my ever-resourceful dad suggested that we just bungee-cord a cardboard box onto the walker. Alas, by this time my friend had run out of time, and we scratched the project. I'd eat my dinner standing at the kitchen counter if necessary; if I wanted to read a book I'd toss it from one end of my tiny apartment to my bed. I'd give the cane, which only required one hand, a whirl.

Despite being somewhat maniacally focused on the basket logistics, I remember riding home through the Saturday afternoon traffic feeling awash with gratitude. I had showed up. The surgeon had done the seemingly miraculous job of fitting me out with a new hip. After months of pain and uncertainty, I was free. I was healthy and alive. I was out. I was one of the lucky ones: I was going home!

My friend got me up to my apartment and more or less settled—not too complicated as basically it came down to choosing whether I'd rather sit in the chair or climb up onto my raised platform bed. I chose the chair.

After she left, I plowed through some piles of mail that had been accumulating since my subtenant left at the end of August. Then, as dusk approached, I tried preparing a meal from the vast stock of Fresh Direct provisions I'd preordered. Alas, the drug-induced nausea prevailed, and most of the food went untouched.

Instead, I turned to Netflix to distract me until I was tired enough (and it was dark enough outside) to sleep. This afternoon set the tone for the days to come, which looking back are a blur of not-quite-sleep narcotic drowsiness and constant nausea, punctuated by occasional restlessness and unpredictable perkiness. The main feeling, recalling my years with bouts of Epstein-Barr virus, was of being an unnoticed recluse, a ghost-like eavesdropper on the rush of life happening in the city all around me.

CHAPTER SEVEN

# THE *REAL* PT BEGINS!

I have no memory of my first visitor. Zero. Zippo.

Somebody—the hospital? The surgeon? My health insurance company?—requires that registered nurses check in on recently released patients to be sure they haven't slipped in the tub, tumbled down the elevator shaft , or otherwise fallen through the cracks.

I only know my nurse came at all because, sensitive to my solitary state and just a tad concerned about my drug-induced welfare, I called Visiting Nurses on Monday morning to ask why no one had come. The startled voice on the other end checked their records and confirmed that someone had indeed paid a visit.

My next official visitor (after the phantom nurse) was my in home physical therapist, Rose. My health insurance company, assuming hip-op graduates will not be terribly mobile to start with, and thus at peril of wandering the streets of New York and/or maneuvering in and out of taxis, entitled me to five home visits.

As with the hospital PT, I was surprised how little she asked of me. All I remember is a brief stroll down the carpeted hallway outside my door, walker and then cane in hand. Clearly we were dealing with baby steps (no pun intended), and I was doing my best to behave, to understand her caution. I failed to mention to her, however, that I was already taking half-hour walks around the neighborhood. (At that point, I'm pretty sure my instructions were not to leave the apartment.) It was September, the weather was glorious, and my apartment depressingly dark and lonely. So out I went, cane in hand. I never did get the hang of using a cane, which seemed to me more of an impediment than an aid to walking. However, my second PT insisted that I carry it with me for weeks after the surgery, if for no other purpose than to signal to others to give me a wide girth. The one thing you *don't* want to do after a hip op is fall and dislocate the implant. The risk of people bumping into you is considerable in New York City. It worked. I traveled in my own little energy bubble, an invisible safety zone, as people bowed wide around me wherever I went.

In fact, it occurred to me that if I really wanted to keep people at a distance, I could circle the cane in the air like a high-school baton twirler, swinging in wide circles this way and that. Except I never was a twirler, and it's a lot harder than it looks.

One sweet thing about these solitary strolls was that I got reacquainted with my neighborhood. I spend so much time out in East Hampton that I have come to think of my New York apartment as my office/yoga studio and my forays into the Big Apple as business trips. So I rarely step out to savor the things that attracted me to the city in the first place—like the bizarre mix of people not witnessed in any other city I've visited around the globe.

And I do love the West Village, maybe because it reminds me of Georgetown, the only semi-urban residential area I knew from growing up in D.C. I've enjoyed watching the area transform. When I arrived in the late 80s, I found hard-core gay culture (I live on Christopher Street, one block down from Stonewall, so think Boots and Saddles, "adult video" stores that double as sex clubs, storefronts of S&M paraphernalia), oddly coupled with staid establishments like Pierre Deux Antiques and fusty, pricey, mediocre restaurants. Now it's a haven of (still way too pricey) designer storefronts. (One designer has so many outlets, we call it Marc Jacobsville.) We get pre-trend things like Japanese roasted-green-tea "espresso" bars and Swedish candy stores that later sprout up elsewhere. There may no longer be lines around the block waiting for cupcakes from Magnolia Bakery, but the establishment appears to still be going strong. Chic tourists tote souvenir shopping bags while posing for selfies. Jo Malone replaced the deli on the ground floor of my building, signaling the sad end of all-night deliveries and the yummy smell of baking chocolate drifting up through the courtyard each morning. Then there is the revolving display of empty storefronts where the rent has pushed out the old guard and mafia owners await those who can pay top dollar for a spot adjacent to Ralph Lauren or Intermix. What started in the newly hip Meat Packing District blew down Bleecker Street, carrying a wave of high-end cool cats (think Williamsburg or Bushwick types endowed with a permanent influx of venture capital). Add in the High Line, the Standard Hotel, and now the new Whitney Museum, and it's a perfect storm of style. I still remember the first time I stood perusing the produce at Gourmet Garage alongside a young woman dressed head to toe in Prada and realized it was time to stop wearing my pajamas to run errands.

Anyway, my second visit from Rose took an unexpected turn. Doing my best to respect her expertise, I asked her if it was okay that I was already doing some yoga (this was probably Day 5 post-op). She asked me what I had in mind, so I dutifully demonstrated a sun salutation. About halfway through, she shut down the laptop where she took notes on my progress and declared, "We're done here."

Huh?

"I can't justify home visits to your insurance company anymore," she finished, "You need to move on." And thus ended our budding relationship. Which, given my limited social intercourse at the time, induced an unexpected wave of sadness.

We spent the rest of that brief visit arranging for my off-site physical therapy. I had already made an appointment for the following week at one of the facilities on my insurance list. However, I am eternally grateful to Rose for nixing that and instead directing me to Infinity Sports Medicine, and specifically to Alex Morales. This tiny storefront operation, wedged between a massage parlor and a restaurant in Chelsea, just in the shadow of Bed Bath and Beyond, became the true Mecca of my healing. Alex is an ex-football player almost twice my size and at least four times as strong, who clearly doesn't believe in wasting anyone's time (i.e., that was the end of my coddling).

After some luscious hands-on work, we'd get down to the business of rebooting my stiff, weak body, which had gotten happily accustomed to lying around most of the day and atrophied accordingly. It's fair to say I didn't know what hit me once Alex started calling the shots. My previous forays into PT had left scant impressions: I remember quitting after my 2001 bike accident because I could tell that what we were doing to heal my elbow fracture was not worth the walk across town. When I had my hand reworked (seven months before the hip surgery) to fix a congenital disease that was bending one finger at an increasingly alarming angle, PT consisted mainly of sitting across the table from my therapist, who spent most of the session giving me a manicure-salon style hand massage. (I do remember glancing over my shoulder at the other poor slobs in the room, who were recovering from knee, hip, and shoulder surgeries, and feeling bad about how hard they were working.)

Let it be said that I pride myself on my physical strength. I'm proud because while naturally flexible, I am not naturally strong. At just over 100 pounds, I've conscientiously built my body into a matrix of lean, sinewy muscle (which may explain while even at my age, I can match 20-year-olds bite-for-bite on daily food consumption and regularly consume about four times as much as people twice my size in my age group). So many of my students have commented on my surprising strength that I've taken on the Altoids mints moniker, "Curiously Strong."

So it was a personal setback to feel weak all over. I never felt like I could manage what Alex asked of me—*ever*—in the many weeks and then months that we worked together. (Sleeping on one side for months to protect the new hip led to a shoulder problem that required a new series of visits, which led to a discovery of scoliosis . . . and so on.) As much as I enjoyed Alex's company, I came to dread our sessions and tried to avoid glancing up at the clock during the toughest maneuvers, only to be discouraged that so little time had passed. When I later expressed my frustration that I always felt like I was letting Alex down because I couldn't do it all, he sweetly (and I hope sincerely!) replied, "But Lois, that's because I give you the stuff no one else can do—you're Superwoman!"

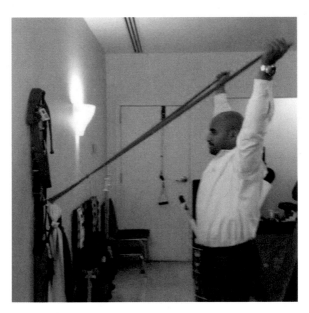

So what did we do? Lots of walking up and down the hallway with Therabands wrapped around my ankles to strengthen my outer hips, hamstrings, and quads. We walked forward. We walked backward. We walked sideways. We walked in a sitting-down posture putting all the weight in my heels to fire up my hamstrings and glutes. We took giant lunges forward and back to restore stability. We stood on a squishy pad and then a wobble board to test my balance. In the beginning Alex would hold my shoulders so I didn't fall. Then one day I noticed he was pushing me side to side and front to back, deliberately throwing me off balance to see if/how I recovered. We did leg lifts and knee-straightening, occasionally (but rarely) on a seated machine where Alex could keep upping the resistance. We went down on all fours with weights behind my knee and did leg lifts. And more stuff I'd prefer to forget.

Then I'd hobble home with an iPhone full of photos of stuff to practice at home. Sometimes if I was really shot I'd take the subway two stops from 18<sup>th</sup> Street to Christopher and flop down on my bed when I arrived.

About those photos: insurance authorized 12 post-op visits, three times a week for four weeks, 30 minutes each session, with, I believe, an option to renew. Being basically unemployed (I couldn't demonstrate for or adjust my private yoga clients in New York City; I couldn't drive to get to my group classes in the Hamptons), I had plenty of time on my hands. And a strong motivation to get back on two feet as soon as possible.

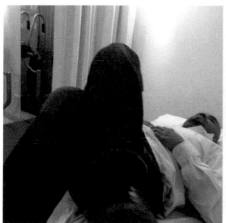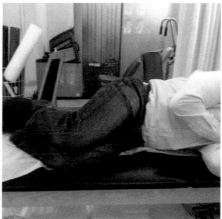

I will say that I lucked out in finding Alex. Not all PTs are equally well trained, experienced, and passionate about what they do. So while it might seem awkward to switch midstream, and your insurance company might offer limited options, you should take this phase of recovery seriously. If you feel for any reason that your PT is not up to the job, not moving you along, or just not a good fit, I urge you to shop around. The right person is out there. Ask doctors, hospitals, friends, massage therapists and bodyworkers, athletes, and anyone you know who's been through a similar injury or surgery for people they liked. Your window for optimal healing is brief (before the scar tissue solidifies and your muscles start compensating for each other in unfortunate ways), so take the actions needed to keep you on the best path.

## STICKING WITH IT

Let nobody tell you that rehab is fun, interesting, or inspiring. In fact, most of the time it's dispiriting to acknowledge that your body just can't do stuff it used to do with ease. It can be frustrating to hit plateaus or sense that you're not progressing. Most of the time, it's just plain boring.

So how to stick with it?

To me it was all about *why*. I wanted to be back in full form. I couldn't accept that halfway through my life I'd be so compromised. Maybe that was just too scary.

I also set an unrealistic deadline for my recovery (more on that below) that involved a commitment to others, so I was duty-bound to get up and at it.

Also, PT is when you get to step up to the plate. The surgeons have done their thing; your time as passive patient is over. You get to actively participate in your recuperation. How much do you care about your recovery? At this point it's largely up to you.

If you don't have a concrete goal looming on the horizon, make one up. Plan a trip. Sign up for a fitness challenge. Schedule a work project that requires that you be mobile. Psychologists call this "good stress," and unlike the nasty, Cortisol-inducing "bad stress," it's actually good for you. If in doubt, picture a life with no goals, no deadlines, no hurdles to leap over, nothing to strive for. Now *that's* depressing.

First I would draw what we did and go home to practice it—only to discover my drawings were basically indecipherable. The iPhotos produced much more satisfying results. I'd go home and practice for an hour or more each day. I still remember the day it occurred to me that my building's security cameras were probably capturing my Theraband sideways crab walks up and down the fourth-floor corridor. Or my stomping up and down the fire stairs with an 8-pound weight wrapped around my right ankle. During this time they were repairing the garbage chute, and I befriended a guy whose dismal job entailed hanging out in the darkened staircase for hours on end. He'd cheer me on as I lugged my slow leg up and down countless flights of stairs.

But I was beyond caring. I was willing to do whatever it took, however ridiculous it might look to others. When I finally made it back out to East Hampton, my housemates soon got used to my pacing up and down the living room, bound legs and all. By this point, I'd gotten so adept—and so bored with—the moves that I often had a book or magazine in hand and read my way through the torture. No reason to let my mind atrophy along with my body!

Besides, we had this deadline looming. Exactly eight weeks from the day of my surgery, I was scheduled to fly to Beijing and then Shenzhen (in southern China) to lead two yoga teacher trainings—seven hours a day, seven days a week for a month straight. While my doctor and travel agent seemed most concerned about whether I'd be okay sitting for the 14-hour flight, I had bigger doubts.

First of all, I had failed to alert my Chinese hosts of my surgical adventure, being fairly certain that if I did, they would cancel the trip. Second, (how) was I going to lead and demonstrate four hours of advanced yoga practice every day, which usually includes many acrobatic moves? These included:

- Full backbend ("wheel" in yoga speak).
- Inversions like a one-handed handstand and a forearm balance with my legs crossed in full lotus.
- Deep, seated hip openers (pre-op torture).
- Standing poses of all sorts, especially the balancing on one leg kind.
- Too many arm and hand balances to name or describe here.

Add to this, my trainings include sessions on hands-on adjustments that require my full strength and stability, not to mention the ability and agility to:

- Get down on hands and knees to delve into students' knotty hip flexors, hamstrings, shoulders, and more.
- Sit or stand back to back with a student while I swing him or her over my shoulder to stretch tight chest muscles.
- Stand in "water ski" position and pull on a strap to lengthen a student's spine (holding so tight that if they release, I go flying backwards).
- Stabilize students with my hands and knees as they attempt to kick or jump up into handstand.

You get the picture. So whenever I flagged, or Alex caught that discouraged look in my eyes, he'd chant our mantra: "China! China! China!" Even my surgeon got with the program, sizing me up at my four-week post-op visit (we moved it back from six weeks to be sure I was ahead of schedule) and predicting I'd be fine halfway around the globe.

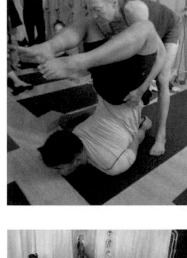

Optimism, like all emotions, is contagious, and I was soon confident that I could in fact pull off the China Odyssey.

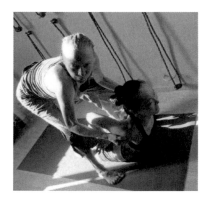

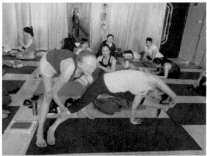

CHAPTER EIGHT

## CHINA LIFTOFF!

The day finally arrived (November 8, I believe), when I would board the plane for the 14-hour flight to Beijing. Let it be said going into this adventure that I do not travel light, and I could already foresee how this might complicate matters.

For example, while I could easily ride a bike the two miles from my house in East Hampton to the beach, this has proved pretty much impossible. My brief excursions to the beach require a small armory of equipment and supplies, including:

- Beach towel and beach umbrella (awkward to place cross-wise over the handle bars, though trust me, I've tried).
- Beach hat, layers of SPF clothing to be worn on the beach and in the water.
- Extra sweaters of various weights for nippy days.
- Multiple water bottles kept in a cooler (I tend to run hot and drink all day, every day).
- Reading material: Never sure what I'll crave at any moment, this usually includes a novel, a serious nonfiction book I've been meaning to tackle for months (and come to think of it rarely if ever do read at the beach), a serious magazine (*Foreign Affairs, The Economist*), a frivolous magazine (fashion or one of the ubiquitous Hamptons summer freebies), and copies of the two local newspapers (highly impractical as the wind blows them every which way like sails, filling the folds with sand in the process and making reading pretty much impossible).
- Sunscreen for my body, sunscreen for my hair, earplugs (to keep water out of my ears), makeup in case I am heading somewhere afterward and need to look presentable (despite wet hair, damp clothes, and sand between my toes).
- Business papers and pens for when I'm justifying my beach time as work time. Back in the day when I worked as an editor, at least one puzzled employer asked why he found sand between the sheets of a manuscript I submitted!

Similarly, when I travel back and forth every week between East Hampton and New York City, I'm always baffled by those ladies on the Hampton Jitney carrying just a handbag. When my parents first bought the house in East Hampton, friends advised me to cut down on the schlepping by buying two of everything I use daily: one set for East Hampton, one for the city. I dutifully doubled up on toiletries, vitamins, prescriptions, sneakers, sandals, yoga pants and tops, sweaters, jackets, water bottles, and reading material. Thing is, with my luckless combination of ADD and general forgetfulness, I inevitably find myself with two of one thing in one place and none in the other. This has particularly wrought havoc on my grocery shopping: I'll arrive to find one fridge practically empty while having left a small garden of produce rotting in the other.

So, as you can imagine, packing for a month-long journey across the planet to a country where I cannot count on getting prescription refills, dental floss, band-aids, nail files, ear plugs, Ibuprophen, alarm clocks, English reading material, computer chargers, cell phone accessories, or any number of daily amenities due to unreliable translations and cultural differences (do the Chinese floss??) requires seemingly endless foresight, countless lists, and a good 10 days of planning. I also take herbal tinctures prescribed by my alternative doctor, 2-oz glass bottles that, depending on the length of my visit, can number as high as 30 and have to be packed in sturdy boxes to avoid breakage.

Food is also an issue. While I've streamlined my visits over ten years of travel to China, sending ahead a list of food to be stocked for my arrival, I can never count on what gets lost in translation as my eager Chinese hosts do their best to meet my requests. Carrying fresh produce is of course verboten on international travel, as every country has its paranoia about germs and insects arriving with foreign guests. So I stock up on dried sea vegetables that miraculously blossom when soaked in boiling water, freeze-dried soup mixes, canned tuna, crackers, and protein bars in case I arrive late at night to an empty fridge—or no fridge at all. Plus, since most of my Chinese "kitchens" are makeshift hotel rooms supplied with a stove top, maybe microwave oven, and an electric tea kettle, it's rare that I will also find mixing bowls, soup bowls, plates, cups, or utensils. Usually it's one undersized soup/tea bowl and a pair of chopsticks. So into my bag go knife, fork, and spoon; plastic bowl and plate; and American-style oversized coffee mug.

All of which pretty much requires a suitcase of its own.

If I'm lucky, I'll arrive to find an array of fruit, vegetables, eggs, and fish or duck that more or less resembles my list. But there are always surprises. One host, one of only two vegans total whom I have met in my 20 journeys around China, tacitly refuses to supply me with any animal protein, leaving my hypoglycemic body on a carbohydrate high that makes me jittery and unfocused. Much to my dismay, the Chinese also have no concept of salad. The closest thing I've ever received was an anemic head of iceberg lettuce, which my hosts most likely diligently foraged from one of the few supermarkets catering to Westerners. When traveling during the summer months or in the semitropical southern regions, I crave cool, raw food. Alas, I'm often treated to sizeable bags of rice and beans and vegetables like sweet potatoes, a weird bamboo-like green vegetable that's about 97% fiber, and other items only edible after substantial boiling, simmering, or sautéing. And then there's the ever puzzling selection of fruits, many of which, as far as I can tell, carry no English names or equivalents. My personal favorites: a green and pink, spiky blimp with a tasteless white and black-seeded interior (I later looked this up and believe it's called dragon fruit) and a melon whose noxious smell permeates whole towns each spring when sold by the outdoor vendors lining many streets. I've never actually sampled that one. As one of my translators put it, "If you don't like the smell, you won't like the taste."

I've survived some trips on a relentless diet of bananas and hard-boiled eggs.

I'm also traveling for work, which means another suitcase devoted to anatomy books, philosophy books, yoga books, and handouts. I bring gifts for my hosts, my translators, my assistants, the studio owners, and anyone else who will inevitably care for me in my helplessly monolingual state. And my yoga brochures. And cards that I make for graduates of my programs. And photographs of myself for the same, to avert the inevitable Chinese photo-thon at the close of each program, during which everyone wants a photo with "teacher," with teacher and this friend, teacher and that friend, teacher and

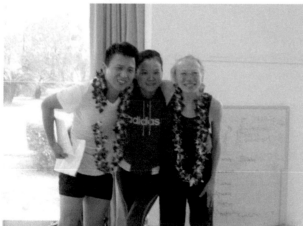

translator, teacher and host . . . you get the picture. And given smart phones' instant feedback loop, most of these photos have to be retaken because their subjects don't like the way they come out. I have left these sessions, which can go on for hours, with my smile muscles nearly paralyzed and my neck kinked from leaning into my Chinese students, most of whom stand a good head shorter than I.

And then of course I need to carry enough yoga clothes to appear if not affluent, at least respectably solvent. (I have long suspected that my Chinese students assume that I am some kind of superstar teacher in the West, and given what they put out to train with me, I am loath to dissuade them of this view.) However, washing machines are still a bit of a rarity in China, which means I am often hand-washing my clothes. Dryers are pretty much unheard of, so once washed, my clothes drape over chairs, tables, desks, headboards, shower rods, and any other suspendable surfaces in hopes that they will dry—*sometime*. Many places I have traveled in China are extremely humid, and it can literally take days for clothes to dry. More than once I have packed soggy shirts, shorts, and pants into suitcases in time to travel to the next city. Which then means that upon arrival I am also carrying soggy books and papers that were nestled into the same bag—all adding to my total kilos of luggage.

In general when traveling to China, I break my iron-clad rule of never bringing more than I can carry—a habit instilled in me from years of traveling in and out of New York City, where one repeatedly encounters subway staircases, a dearth of taxis, and other scenarios in which if you can't haul your own stuff, you're simply out of luck. China-bound, I am burdened with enough stuff to sustain a small family for months.

So I was skeptical that November that I would make it to through airport check-ins, as well as in and out of various cars and taxis, and up and down hotel or studio staircases loaded down with more than I could carry with two good hips. But by now I was accustomed to assuming the role of damsel in distress (hereafter DID). I shamelessly fussed and fidgeted at curbsides, and security gates, and when boarding or leaving planes, until it was clear to some hapless observer that I needed help. At which point I would explain about my metal hip and usually receive some gracious assistance. I hoped things would get easier as the trip progressed, since I would be eating my way through my food, distributing gifts, cards, and handouts, and downing bottles of herbal tinctures, thus lightening my load. I failed to calculate the additional weight and space occupied by the many sweet and thoughtful gifts my students and hosts bestowed upon me at each venue. Among other more portable mementos, I have returned home from trips with:

- An elegant but extremely heavy mahjong set (if you've never played mahjong, picture a solid wooden box about the size of 2 briefcases, holding a collection of ivory chips a little larger than Scrabble letters).

- A boxed, poster sized image of a Chinese (Buddhist?) diety, complete with wooden frame and two-part explanatory CD in Mandarin that would not play in Western CD players).
- A desktop glass rendering of Xian's 10,000 warriors weighing in about five pounds.
- A glass replica of the Eiffel Tower filled with hundreds of tiny "good luck" origami stars (still puzzling over this one).
- A styrofoam box holding a dozen of my favorite "century eggs," a weirdly delicious Chinese delicacy made by burying eggs deep in lead-rich soil till they age and ferment or undergo some chemical process I have yet to fathom.
- A collection of naked porcelain babies.
- A lovely, large-format calligraphy on rIce paper that required careful rolling to not be squashed (and which, my Japanese assistant later informed me, I had hung upside-down in my New York kitchen).
- Several apparently quite valuable and extremely fragile tea sets.
- A custom-designed, knee-length Maoist jacket.
- Reams of mala beads, necklaces, and earrings.
- Picture books from students' native provinces.
- Yoga books with Mandarin text I will never decipher.

So I was bound to return to New York laden with at least as much as I had brought. A dilemma faced by many seasoned recreational travelers, but one that I could ill afford in my still precarious ambulatory state.

Luckily, my hip surgeon had provided me with a credit-card sized image of a hip implant, with the date inscribed on it, that I was to present at airport security check-ins. The metal implants can set off the security alarms, and this did happen on my way from Beijing to Shenzhen. I was between translators at the time, and unfortunately when the alarm went off, my bag containing the card was itself making its way through the x-ray machine. Unable to convey to the airport staff the source of the problem, I finally flagged down another English-speaking traveler who brought my bag over and enabled me to flash the hip card. God knows how long that encounter might have dragged out otherwise, and whether I might have ended up in some grim, post-Communist detention cell while the authorities ascertained why my body was lighting up its metal detector.

In any case, the hip card proved quite handy. When limping along, or stymied by my burden of baggage, or running late and in need of a quick glide through security, I could pull out the card and pray that airport officials would take pity on a DID and facilitate my passage. I have even considered carrying this card with me *everywhere*, as its applications to a broad range of pickles gradually dawned on me.

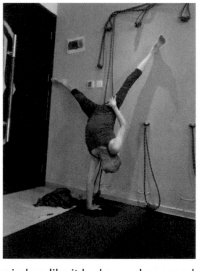

Luckily again, the gods were with me on my new hip's maiden voyage to the land of the future. My hip held up through an impressive amount of schlepping. It adapted to sitting still for the long overseas flight with only a little residual stiffness. And miracle of miracles, I found I was able to sail through the long days of teaching with only minor discomfort.

I must say that my hosts and translator were a little baffled, not to say chagrined, that I had not shared the news of my surgery with them. Once over this awkward hurdle, however, we carried on like it had never happened.

Each day as I led yoga practices and did my share of demonstrating, my confidence grew. Since I had been mainly focusing back home on my physical therapy exercises and not on pushing the limits of my yogic flexibility and strength, it was refreshing to see how quickly I was back in the saddle. Within a week I was up to my usual tricks—wacky arm balances, deep backbends, dicey balances.

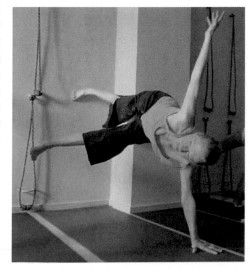

About this time I emailed my surgeon two especially remarkable feats: a one-handed handstand in which the other hand is "shaking hands" with a student, and an upside-down pose in which my weight is on my forearms while

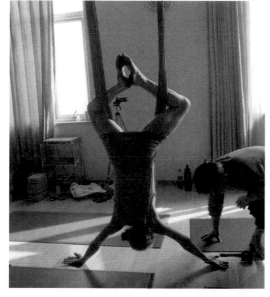

my legs are crossed in full lotus. Inversions aside, I had not been able to do anything like a lotus, seated, upside down, or otherwise, for months before my surgery. I cheerfully attached a brief note below the photos stating: "I hope you understand that I'm not doing anything I consider risky!" To which he replied, "Fantastic! Enjoy the rest of your trip." The following September, when I went in for my one-year post-op exam, he did admit to being a bit concerned about my intrepid approach to recovery.

Those photos and others from that same trip took an interesting journey of their own through the HSS email hierarchy. Convinced by that point that my apparently astonishing recovery might inspire other patients, I asked

whether I might assist HSS in their publicity campaigns. My surgeon's assistant concurred and suggested that I forward the China photos to their PR team, who were planning the next year's advertising campaign. While I had already written a brief text and supplied photos for "Back in the Game," HSS's website feature of patients happy with their results, we both thought my case deserved more attention. After I forwarded the photos, a long silence

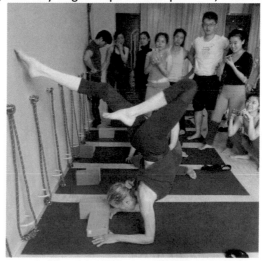

ensued. Eventually it occurred to me that my progress was just possibly *too* off the charts. Somewhere deep in "don't try this at home" territory. A potential source of litigation if other patients assumed they'd be engaging in the same acrobatics after surgery. So instead I funneled my energy into this book, where the photos are placed in their rightful context as evidence of how I was able to return to my optimal pre-op activities, not become something I had never been before.

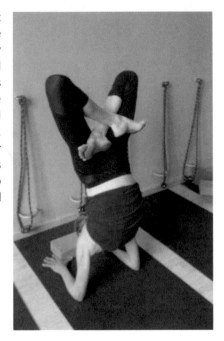

CHAPTER NINE

# The Home Stretch

That trip to China was really the turning point, or the last bend in the road of my journey from cripple to rehab to life as normal as mine will ever be.

That said, a couple of annoying, though not unworkable, after-effects emerged in the following months. Having been told not to sleep on my right side for at least three months, preferably longer, I slept all night, every night, on my left side. And as I was recovering, I was sleeping or at least resting a *lot*. I am left-handed and totally left dominant, and putting all of my upper body weight on a rounded left shoulder during the night tightened up that joint like a screw. Throbbing pain that traveled from my shoulder to my elbow woke me up throughout the night, every night.

So, I was back to the PT for another few months of work to unravel the collateral damage. It appears that those months of sideways bedrest were the final straw in a lifetime of overworking my left arm and shoulder. A long-distance swimmer in the days before we were taught to breathe out of alternate sides, I had cultivated a rounded left shoulder through right-side-only breathing during thousands of miles up and down countless pools. A perpetual student before the age of laptops, I also spent 25 years of schooling taking fastidious notes with that shoulder rounded forward and down, often in a cross-body position to conform to those right-handed plastic chair-and-desk combos that cleverly place the "desk" surface well to the right. And of course, that being my stronger arm, I carried my backpack and bags on that side; I lifted and carried and pushed and pulled everything with my left arm.

Four years post-hip op, that shoulder still bothers me. I'd love to be able to report that PT did the job, or even that another surgery restored my left shoulder to optimal flexibility and strength as it had my hip. But the shoulder is a complicated joint, with surgical outcomes and rehab success far from assured. No one, not my doctors or my PT or anyone else I consulted, thought I should go that route. So we're in a holding pattern on that front.

Related to, and perhaps resulting from, the shoulder asymmetry and months of limping, my PT also discovered a sideways curve in my lower back. I was not born with scoliosis and did not develop it during the typical teenage growth spurt. The standard supine X-ray does not show the curve. However, HSS uses a stand-up X-ray machine for imaging hips, and there it was obvious that when weight bearing I both lean and twist to the right. So, more PT to address that.

Finally, about a year after my hip op, I noticed a disturbingly familiar pain in my *left* hip. Exactly where the pain had begun on the other side. People often ask when you say you are going in for or have had hip surgery, "One or both?" History has borne out that those who lose one hip eventually lose the other. Arthritis being an equal-opportunity affliction, it's usually just a matter of time before the second hip gives out, and an increasing number of patients decide just to have both done at the same time and get it over with. My left hip did indeed show serious arthritis, but the space between the femur and its socket was considerably larger than on the right, and I felt no pain on that side. Moreover, rehabbing and generally getting through the day with one functional hip is considerably easier than with none. Since I could not afford full-time custodial care and none of my relatives or loved ones was available to provide the same, bilateral surgery was in any case not an option for me.

But when hip number two started to act up, I immediately jumped to (or sank to) the devastating conclusion that I was on my way to hip op number two. I started projecting increasing pain, reduced range of motion, hobbling about, the seemingly endless string of visits to doctors, X-rays and MRIs, surgical consults, insurance hijinks, and eventual surgery. I'd lie awake at night mapping out when I would be able to clear my schedule for another surgery and rehab. I calculated costs and pondered how I'd cope with additional debt. Things got very dark inside.

About that time, I went in for my one-year post-op visit with my surgeon. He was delightfully reassuring and characteristically optimistic, informing me that my X-rays showed no deterioration in the left hip since the first surgery. Instead, he prescribed more PT, focusing on releasing the muscles that were over-working and strengthening those that had apparently gone slack.

I went back to Alex. We spent a few sessions puzzling our way through what was going on. My first guess was that I had overdone the "crab walk" exercise in which Therabands wrapped around my ankles sent my abductor muscles into overdrive. That path led nowhere. Somewhere around the fourth visit we figured out that it wasn't my hip but my lower back that was causing the problem. A muscle called the quadratus lumborum, a rectangle strung between the bottom ribs and the top of the pelvis, was the culprit.

Called the "hip hiker," the QL when engaged only on one side raises that hip. Well, now that I was sleeping *only* on my right side to protect my left shoulder, the left QL was passively contracted all night. Once we got it stretched out (and I resumed occasionally sleeping on the left side), the problem went away. Whew!

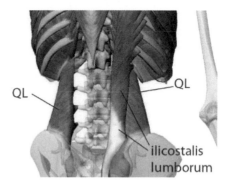

*Source: loveyogaanatomy.com*

Beyond that, the aftermath of my hip op lingers on other fronts. On the positive side, I have become an informal counselor to many considering or recovering from hip replacements. I renewed my dedication to helping anyone, anywhere to cope with or heal from structural (physical) problems that I trust I understand. I've been motivated to write this book to widen my scope of inspiration and influence beyond my immediate circle and the various individuals who have found their way into my inbox or my voicemail.

The downside: my pool of group-class and private yoga students dwindled during the months before my surgery, plummeted to zero for a brief period afterward, and took awhile to return to pre-op levels. It's true that many of my current students have been drawn to me *because* they know what I have been through and how deeply I care about helping others. But the dip, however temporary, had a huge impact on my professional life (see "PR Nightmare") above. It's just possible that an equal number of students have shied away from me, reasonably concluding that a yoga teacher who ends up needing hip surgery clearly doesn't know what she's doing. (I have heard through the grapevine of several yoga teachers far more famous than I who have chosen to conceal the fact that they have undergone hip, knee, or shoulder surgeries, I can only assume due to this same concern.)

The reduced income topped with medical expenses left a wake of debt. While on a good day I can always remind myself, "It's only money; at least you have your health," credit card companies, landlords, utility providers, and others are much less interested in my wellbeing than they are in the bottom line. I wake up daily and go to bed each night with that burden.

However, the sum total of this journey has been my emergence as one confident, buoyant, and eternally grateful individual. Not a day goes by when I do not realize what a wonder it is that I can walk down the sidewalk without pain, that I can climb stairs like a normal person (even going up two at a time to challenge my strength), that I can walk the soft, uneven sandy beach on summer mornings for an hour or more without pain.

6 MONTHS POST-OP

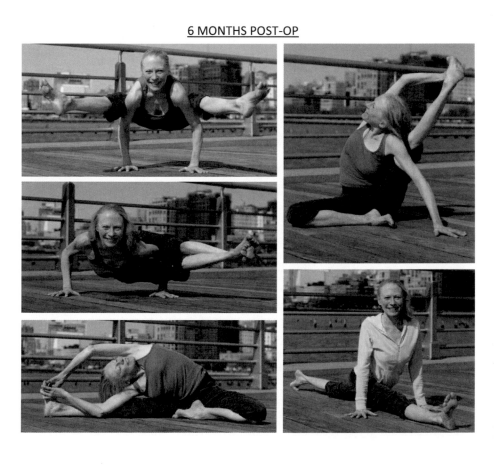

How does one end a happy story? How can I express my gratitude without spawning envy in those less fortunate than I? How can I avoid sounding smug if not invincible?

I can only hope that no one reads this final chapter without reading all that led me to where I am today. I can only hope that by sharing my trials and triumphs, my fears and my courage, my doubts and my resolve—all offered by a woman who got through a tough situation with a fortunate mix of luck, love, and spirit—others will be stirred to action. That they, or "you," dear reader, will face whatever life has thrown your way with:

- Trust in yourself
- Faith in the universe
- And a willingness to take the next right step at every stage of your journey

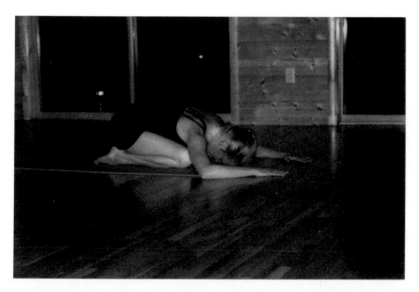

As the Arab saying goes, "Pray to Allah, but tie up your camel." In other words, fuse hope with common sense, faith with action. Don't go it alone, but don't expect God or the universe to do it all for you. Fuse the two, and I believe that you will find within yourself and the world around you all that you need to prevail. You may not be restored to perfect health. You may not heal a broken relationship. You may forever grieve the loss of a loved one. You may never bounce back from a layoff or other career debacle. On the other hand, you may. You may cross over to the other side.

I'd like to end with a modification I've made to the classic Buddhist meditation known as *metta*, or lovingkindness. In this practice, one begins by repeating the same phrases over and over again silently to oneself:

May I be safe
May I be happy
May I be healthy
May I live with ease.

To me, that's a somewhat overwhelming list of requests/demands. There are still plenty of days, or at least plenty of moments in many days, when fear's nimble fingers grab hold of me and I feel anything *but* safe. I come undone at the prospect of a difficult conversation, a mysterious physical symptom, the prospect of long-term insolvency. I can wallow in the darkness as well as the next guy or gal, retreat to my cave, delving deep into the many shades of sad, glum, melancholy, and disconsolate till I forget that "happy" is even on the spectrum. Thanks to a fragile immune system, at times you could knock me over with a feather, and my hours of bouncing-ball energy can easily be matched by afternoon naps and other prolonged sleep-ins as I wait around to feel better. And as for living with ease, I seem to have been born a struggler. Life as one perpetual challenge (and at times chore) is part of my DNA. When my first psychiatrist asked why I couldn't just be more "laid back," I had this image of the world falling apart around me. I'm weighed down by responsibilities you can't even imagine—and come to think of it, neither can I. I just know that something truly tremendous depends on my never letting up. You take the easy path; I'll be up in the watchtower making sure you're safe.

So continuing to fail pretty much daily at these four requests, I've narrowed the agenda down to a short form that's good enough to get me through the average day:

*May I be.*

I'll take life with negative net worth across my bank accounts. I'll face heartbreak and live with sorrow. I'll accept one good hip. I'll take on each day as an uphill battle with miles to go before I sleep. I'll never lose sight of my belief that life in *any* form is a gift. It's a privilege to be here. It's a privilege to *be*.

Of course I'll do what I can to alleviate suffering—my own and that of anyone and everyone, including animals and plants and our blessed planet. But I've also been humbled enough to know that that project is greater than the resources of one little human. So I'll continue to start and end each day with one simple prayer:

*May I be.*

*Lois Nesbitt*

*May 2018*

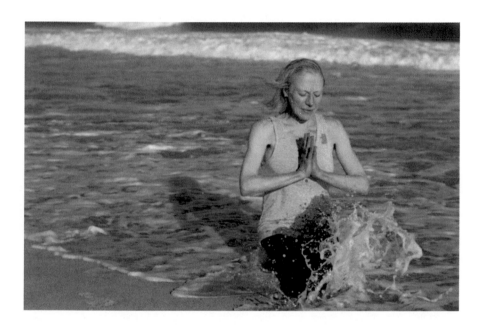

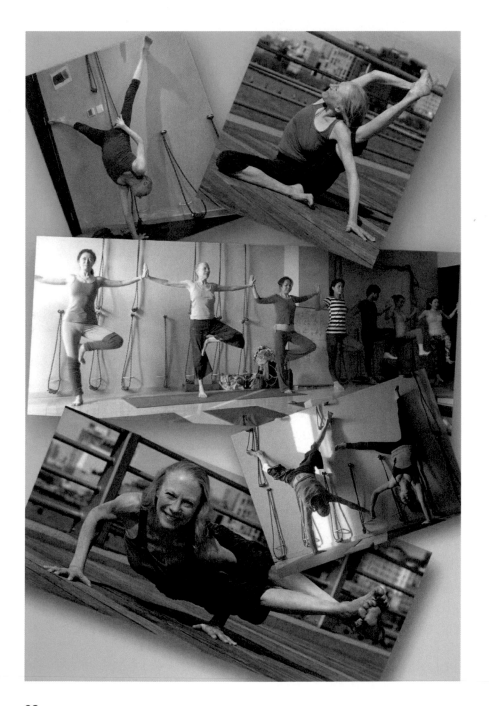

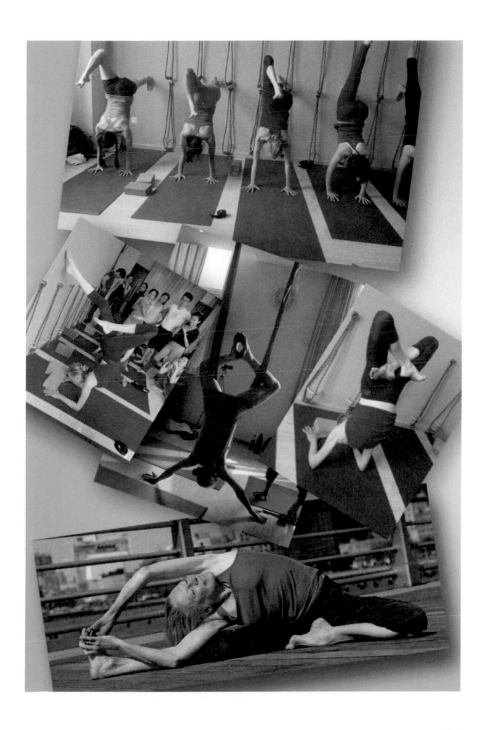

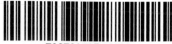

Made in the USA
Middletown, DE
26 September 2019